Neurological Rehabilitation of Parkinson's Disease

Neurological Rehabilitation of Parkinson's Disease

Edited by
Diane Playford MD FRCP
Senior Lecturer
Institute of Neurology, University College London
and Honorary Consultant in Neurology,
National Hospital for Neurology and Neurosurgery,
University College London Hospitals Trust,
Queen Square, London, UK

Series Editor
Alan J Thompson MD FRCP FRCPI
Garfield Weston Professor of Clinical
Neurology and Neurorehabilitation
Institute of Neurology, University College London
and Honorary Consultant in Neurology,
National Hospital for Neurology and Neurosurgery,
University College London Hospitals Trust,
Queen Square, London, UK

MD **Martin Dunitz**
Taylor & Francis Group
LONDON AND NEW YORK

BS

First published in the United Kingdom in 2003
by Martin Dunitz, an imprint of the Taylor & Francis Group, 11 New Fetter Lane,
London EC4P 4EE

Tel.:   +44 (0) 20 7583 9855
Fax.:   +44 (0) 20 7842 2298
E-mail: info@dunitz.co.uk
Website: http://www.dunitz.co.uk

A CIP record for this book is available from the British Library.

ISBN 1 84184 297 4

Distributed in the USA by
Fulfilment Center
Taylor & Francis
10650 Tobben Drive
Independence, KY 41051, USA
Toll Free Tel.: +1 800 634 7064
E-mail: taylorandfrancis@thomsonlearning.com

Distributed in Canada by
Taylor & Francis
74 Rolark Drive
Scarborough, Ontario M1R 4G2, Canada
Toll Free Tel.: +1 877 226 2237
E-mail: tal_fran@istar.ca

Distributed in the rest of the world by
Thomson Publishing Services
Cheriton House
North Way
Andover, Hampshire SP10 5BE, UK
Tel.: +44 (0)1264 332424
E-mail: salesorder.tandf@thomsonpublishingservices.co.uk

Printed and bound in Great Britain by The Cromwell Press, Trowbridge, Wilts.

10/29/03

Contents

Contributors

Roger A Barker
Cambridge Centre for Brain
    Repair
Forvie Site
Robinson Way
Cambridge CB2 2PY, UK

Kailash P Bhatia
Sobell Department of
    Movement Neuroscience
    and Movement Disorders
Institute of Neurology
University College London
Queen Square
London WC1N 3BG, UK

Maria Bozi
Sobell Department of
    Movement Neuroscience
    and Movement Disorders
Institute of Neurology
University College London
Queen Square
London WC1N 3BG, UK

Katherine Deane
Division of Neuroscience
University of Birmingham
Department of Neurology
City Hospital NHS Trust
Dudley Road
Birmingham B18 7QH, UK

Ray Fitzpatrick
Division of Public Health and
    Primary Health Care

Institute of Health Sciences
University of Oxford
Old Road
Headington
Oxford OX3 7LF, UK

Marjan Jahanshahi
Sobell Department of
    Movement Neuroscience
    and Movement Disorders
Institute of Neurology
University College London
Queen Square
London WC1N 3BG, UK

Simon JG Lewis
Cambridge Centre for Brain
    Repair
Forvie Site
Robinson Way
Cambridge CB2 2PY, UK

Diane Playford
Institute of Neurology
University College London
Queen Square
London WC1N 3BG, UK

Dorothy Robertson
The Older People's Unit
Royal United Hospital
Combe Park
Bath BA1 3NG, UK

Series Preface

Neurological rehabilitation aims to decrease the impact of neurological disorders and minimise their impact on those affected by them. The importance of managing the consequences of acute and chronic neurological disorders is increasingly acknowledged, as is the role that neurologists can and should play in minimising their impact. This has required a broader focus for neurological practice, which, in turn, has a major implication for training.

This series, written by people from a variety of backgrounds, is an attempt to deliver the essentials of neurological rehabilitation in a concise and user-friendly fashion. It will cover a range of neurological disorders all of which have a major impact on those affected. The first in the series describes the management of Parkinson's disease. It brings together a multidisciplinary team of experts and is edited by Dr Diane Playford. It is hoped that by publishing the essential elements in a concise and accessible format it will prove a useful and much used aid in patient management.

Alan J Thompson
Series Editor

Preface

Parkinson's disease (PD) is one of the commonest progressive neurological disorders. In common with other such disorders, there is a growing consensus that it is best managed using a multidisciplinary approach. The physician has a key role in the drug management of PD and this is reflected in Chapter 1, but later chapters consider the impact of the disorder on the patient and family, rehabilitation therapies, service delivery and measurement of outcome. The final chapter considers the potential for recovery and repair.

The randomized controlled trial (RCT) is regarded as the gold standard for evidence-based medicine, and there are many RCTs to demonstrate the role of different dopaminergic drugs. However, some aspects of management – such as the role of rehabilitation therapies and how best to deliver a clinical service – are less amenable to the RCT. As a result the literature in this difficult area is not always conclusive.

The aim of this book is to provide a summary of the evidence about the structure and processes that allow the comprehensive management of a patient with PD. Not all services are alike: some are based at neurological centres while others are in departments for healthcare for the elderly or in the community. All need to be able to cater for the needs of patients at diagnosis and the patient with complex disability. I hope this book will identify some of the approaches to establishing comprehensive PD services and also identify areas where further work needs to be done.

Diane Playford

The Pharmacological Management of Parkinson's Disease

Maria Bozi and Kailash P Bhatia

Introduction

Parkinson's disease (PD) is one of the commonest neurodegenerative diseases and amongst the commonest causes of disability in the elderly.

> About 1% of the population over the age of 65 is affected by Parkinson's disease. This ratio rises to 2% in the population over 80 years of age.[1]

PD is characterised by a triad of motor symptoms, namely bradykinesia, rigidity, resting tremor. Pathologically, it is characterised by a progressive loss of the dopaminergic neurones in the substantia nigra that project into the striatum, resulting in a state of dopamine deficiency in the caudate and putamen. Lack of dopamine is the cause of the main motor symptoms of the disease, which classically involve tremor, rigidity and bradykinesia. It is widely accepted that the pathological process extends beyond the basal ganglia and affects other CNS neuronal populations that utilize other neurotransmitters such as serotonin (raphe nuclei), norepinephrine (locus ceruleus) and acetylcholine (pedunculopontine nucleus). The involvement of these non-dopaminergic pathways is believed to account for the non-motor symptoms of PD, as well as for symptoms that do not respond to dopaminergic medication. These symptoms include postural instability, freezing, alterations of mentation, behaviour and mood, sleep disorders and autonomic dysfunction. The cause of PD is uncertain but both genetic and environmental factors seem to contribute to its pathogenesis in the majority of cases.[1,2]

The management of PD is complex since the clinician has to deal with a chronic and progressively disabling disease with a large spectrum of motor and non-motor symptoms. Superimposed on the symptoms of the disease are early and late side-effects of medication.

Four different clinical stages can be recognized throughout the course of the disease.[3] The first stage of *diagnosis* is followed by the stage of *maintenance* during which a good control of the patient's symptoms is achieved without complications. The *complex stage* is characterized by the presence of complications such as motor fluctuations, dyskinesias and other non-motor symptoms. The last is the *palliative stage* where therapeutic interventions no longer offer adequate symptomatic control and the patient is severely disabled.

The main goal of the palliative stage is to prevent the complications of immobility, to maintain the social integration of the patient and to reduce the psychological distress of the patient and carer. Medical interventions differ between the early (diagnostic and maintenance) and late (complex and palliative) stages of the disease.

Management of Early-stage Disease

At this stage patients are first informed about the diagnosis. Because of the chronic nature of the disease and the disability that it implies the communication of the diagnosis is stressful. Intervention at this stage aims to facilitate the acceptance of the diagnosis and to reduce stress as well as to relieve symptoms. Provision of accurate and sensitive education to patients and their families, support services and the introduction of patients to specialist nurses, when available, are very important to help patients understand the disease and reconcile themselves with their emerging needs and perspectives. Early education programmes, which include informing patients about services and rehabilitation therapies and their roles are essential. These topics are discussed in more detail in Chapters 3 and 4. Pharmacological treatment should ideally aim to prevent the progression of the disease, relieve symptoms and reduce the risk of motor complications.[4,5]

Prevention of Disease Progression

Prevention in PD should slow down, stop or even reverse the process of neuronal death.

> Many factors have been implicated in the pathogenesis of PD including oxidative stress, mitochondrial dysfunction, excitotoxicity, calcium dysregulation and inflammation.[6]

Agents that interfere with any of these factors could potentially provide neuroprotection; several compounds have been tested but no definite conclusions could be drawn. One limitation is the lack of a method to measure neuronal death *in vivo* since it is uncertain how clinical symptoms correlate with the degree of neuronal loss. Moreover, it is difficult to separate symptomatic from neuroprotective effects clinically.[7] Lately, imaging techniques, such as fluorodopa PET and β-CIT SPECT have been used as objective measures of the progression of the disease, but such endpoints are still exploratory.

Potential neuroprotective agents that have been or are being currently tested include:

- vitamin E (tocopherol) and selegiline because of their antioxidant effects;
- riluzole, an inhibitor of glutamine release and remacemide, a glutamine antagonist, both agents that block glutamate-mediated toxicity;
- anti-inflammatory compounds such as cyclooxygenase-2 inhibitors;
- antiapoptotic drugs including the caspase inhibitor minocycline;
- co-enzyme Q, a compound that acts as a cofactor for mitochondrial complex I. Recently, a study has shown a delay in disease progression in early-stage patients who were treated with co-enzyme Q but further studies are required before any conclusions can be drawn.[8]

Selegiline was one of the first drugs to be tested because of its ability to inhibit the MAO-B-mediated metabolism of dopamine and the formation of free radicals. It is also thought to have anti-apoptotic effects. The delay in the need for levodopa that was noticed in one study in the selegiline group (compared with placebo) was initially interpreted as neuroprotection. However, the current conclusion from the clinical trials with selegiline is that the drug has a mild symptomatic effect, enough to delay the need for levodopa.[9,10]

Lately there has been a growing interest in the putative neuro-protective properties of the dopamine agonists.[11] These agonists could provide protection through several mechanisms by inducing:

- levodopa-sparing effect;
- decreased dopamine synthesis, release and metabolism by the activation of dopamine autoreceptors;
- direct antioxidant effects;
- receptor-mediated anti-apoptotic effects;
- inhibition of excitotoxicity mediated by overactivity of the sub-thalamic nucleus.[12]

Several prospective clinical trials have been initiated to assess the putative effect of dopamine agonists on the rate of progression of PD using clinical and imaging endpoints. Both CALM-PD and REAL-PET studies have demonstrated a slower progression of the disease in patients receiving pramipexole or ropinirole, respectively, compared to levodopa.[13,14] However, as discussed above, the design of the trials to show neuroprotection in PD is controversial and the use of SPECT or PET as endpoints is still exploratory.

At present, despite the increasing interest and the growing body of information, there are insufficient data to recommend any specific regimen for neuroprotection.[8]

Initiation of Symptomatic Therapy

As long as no convincing neuroprotective agent is yet available, treatment is considered when symptoms of PD cause functional disability. Functional impairment should be defined on an individual basis because there are different functional implications for different patients depending on age, profession and lifestyle. Once the initiation of treatment has been agreed, the choice of drug becomes the main issue.[15] The goal of the treatment should be to offer good symptomatic control with a reduced risk of late motor complications. Different options are available, as listed in Box 1.1.

Box 1.1   Drugs that could be used as initial therapy in Parkinson's disease

- Dopamine agonists
- Anticholinergics
- Amantadine
- Selegiline
- Standard-release levodopa
- Controlled-release levodopa
- Standard- or controlled-release levodopa + COMT inhibitor

Amongst them, dopamine agonists and levodopa are the ones that give the best control over parkinsonian symptoms.

Levodopa

Levodopa remains the gold standard treatment for PD.[16] Its dramatic clinical effect in PD was first demonstrated in 1967, when high doses were used by Cotzias.[17]

> Levodopa is the immediate precursor of dopamine and its use replaces the endogenous deficient neurotransmitter.

It is absorbed from the duodenum and penetrates to a certain degree the brain through the blood–brain barrier. In the brain it is converted to dopamine by the enzyme dopa decarboxylase, which is located in the remaining dopaminergic terminals and in extradopaminergic glial and neuronal compartments. Levodopa is combined with the peripheral dopa decarboxylase inhibitors benserazide or carbidopa, which inhibit the conversion of levodopa to dopamine peripherally. Peripheral dopaminergic adverse effects, such as nausea, vomiting and postural hypotension, are thus reduced, central delivery is amplified and the dose of levodopa can be decreased. Levodopa has a short plasma half-life of about 60 to 90 minutes.

Levodopa improves, often dramatically, parkinsonian signs and symptoms, functional disability and perhaps even survival.[18,19] The drug is well tolerated with few side-effects, the commonest ones being nausea, postural hypotension and psychiatric symptoms. Following its initiation, there is a period of sustained uncomplicated response – the 'levodopa honeymoon' – although unfortunately the excellent response is not maintained.[20] After several years of treatment, patients begin to experience response fluctuations and dyskinesias, which are very disabling and difficult to treat.

Several presynaptic and postsynaptic mechanisms are believed to be involved in the pathogenesis of motor complications. The most important ones are the pulsatile non-physiological stimulation of the dopaminergic receptors and the subsequent modulation of many downstream neurotransmitter systems.[21,22] The continued loss of dopaminergic nerve-endings associated with the progression of the disease results in the loss of the storage sites of dopamine formed from levodopa. The formation and release of dopamine shifts to non-dopaminergic compartments that lack the vesicular storage apparatus. Thus, formation of dopamine and receptor stimulation oscillates in parallel with plasma and striatal levodopa levels and so the buffering effect is lost. The short plasma half-life of levodopa contributes to the oscillatory non-physiological stimulation of the dopaminergic receptors. It has also been suggested that motor complications might even be primed by the first doses of levodopa.[23] It is postulated that continuous dopaminergic stimulation from the early phase of treatment will reduce the likelihood of developing motor complications. Therefore motor complications could be prevented or delayed by postponing the initiation of levodopa.

However, the role of levodopa for induction of motor complications remains a matter of controversy.[24] Several studies suggest that the degree of the nigrostriatal degeneration and the way dopaminergic agents are administered are the most important determinants of the development of dyskinesias.[25,26] Pulsatile administration of levodopa and the dopamine agonist apomorphine cause dyskinesias and fluctuations while continuous administration can alleviate existing motor complications.[27,28] The dose of levodopa also seems to play a role, as lower doses are associated with a smaller risk of motor complications.[29]

The hypothesis that the pulsatile stimulation produced by immediate-release levodopa might account for the motor complications has led to the development of controlled-release preparations of the drug. However, clinical trials failed to show any difference in motor complication rates between immediate- and controlled-release levodopa after five years of treatment.[30]

Another concern about levodopa is its possible toxicity to nigral neurones.[31] Relevant data are available from studies on animal models and cell cultures but there is no clinical evidence to support this.[32,33]

When introducing L-dopa as initial or supplementary therapy, one can opt for immediate (standard)-release (starting with 50–100 mg three times per day) or controlled (modified)-release preparations (100 mg three times per day).

COMT (catechol-O-methyltransferase) inhibitors

COMT inhibitors are usually used in the management of more advanced disease. Although the addition of carbidopa or benserazide to levodopa increases the amount of drug available to enter the brain, most levodopa is then metabolized in the gut and liver by COMT to an inactive metabolite 3-O-methyldopa. The COMT inhibitory agents tolcapone and entacapone prevent this breakdown, thus prolonging the half-life of levodopa and increasing its transport to the brain to produce dopamine. There is a suggestion that the early combination of levodopa with COMT inhibitors may reduce the risk of dyskinesias although clinical data are still lacking.

> The side-effects of COMT inhibitors include potentiation of dyskinesias, nausea, hypotension, orange discoloration of the urine and sedation.

Chronic tolcapone use can result in diarrhoea, which can be severe; also, liver toxicity has been associated with tolcapone. Because of four cases of fatal toxic hepatitis, tolcapone was withdrawn from the European market in 1998. Hence entacapone is currently the only available COMT inhibitor in the UK. No association between the drug and liver toxicity has been shown and elevations of liver enzymes have not been reported.[34] Entacapone is administered at a dose of 200 mg together with every levodopa dose up to a limit of 1600 mg daily, while tolcapone is given at three daily doses of 100 or 200 mg.

Dopamine agonists

Drugs in this class act directly on dopamine receptors, mimicking the endogenous neurotransmitter although none of them stimulates the full complement of dopamine receptors in the same way as levodopa.

> Dopamine agonists can be classified into ergot (bromocriptine; pergolide; lisuride; cabergoline) and non-ergot derivatives (apomorphine; pramipexole; ropinirole).

There are several theoretical advantages of dopamine agonists over L-dopa. They usually have a long duration of action and they act directly on the dopamine receptors bypassing the degenerating nigrostriatal terminals. Thus, they provide a more stable and physiological stimulation and may help to prevent or reduce motor complications.[35] In addition, they have putative neuroprotective properties as described in the section on neuroprotection.

In clinical practice dopamine agonists have been shown to be efficacious in Parkinson's disease. They were initially introduced as adjuvant therapy in late disease.[36,37] However, the desire to delay the introduction of levodopa led to trials with dopamine agonists used as monotherapy in early PD. Several prospective double-blind controlled trials have demonstrated the efficacy of dopamine agonists as antiparkinsonian agents when used as monotherapy.[38–40] Their beneficial effects can be sustained for more than three years in the average patient. In a study assessing the efficacy of bromocriptine 20% of patients randomized to bromocriptine remained on monotherapy at five years.[41] A recent study comparing ropinirole with levodopa in early PD showed that approximately 50% of patients could be maintained on ropinirole monotherapy for three years and more than 30% for five years.[42] Most importantly, several clinical trials have demonstrated that initiating symptomatic treatment with a dopamine agonist is associated with a significantly reduced risk for development of motor complications, even in those patients who later received levodopa supplementation. Clinical data are available for bromocriptine,[43] ropinirole,[42] pramipexole,[44] cabergoline,[45] and pergolide[46]. It is worthy of note that in most of these trials patients on dopamine agonists had significantly worse disability scores than patients treated with levodopa.

It is not clear what the ideal pharmacological properties of the dopamine agonists are. Most of those currently available are active at the D2 and D3 receptors. It is reasonable to hypothesize that the stimulation of both D1 and D2 class receptors is required for full efficacy. Apomorphine, an agonist, which is administered subcutaneously, has the ability to stimulate both D1 and D2 class receptors and may be more effective at controlling parkinsonian symptoms than the other available agonists. The limitations for its widespread use are its lack of oral bioavailability, short half-life and high incidence of side-effects, such as nausea and local skin reactions at the site of injection. Its continuous subcutaneous infusion is used with good results in fluctuating and dyskinetic patients.[47] Other routes of apomorphine administration are being investigated including nasal and sublingual as well as administration through a portable pump for IV infusion.[48,49]

The half-life of different dopamine agonists is longer than that of levodopa ranging from 6 to 12 hours. Cabergoline is the longest-acting compound. Its half-life of 72 hours allows once-daily dosing. Transdermal patch preparations of a new dopamine agonist (rotigotine), which would allow a stable release of the drug throughout a 24 hour period, are being currently tested for efficacy and tolerability.[50]

> The spectrum of side-effects of dopamine agonists is similar to that of levodopa and includes nausea, vomiting, postural hypotension and somnolence, plus psychiatric side-effects such as confusion, hallucinations and, more rarely, delusional states.

Dopamine agonists have a greater propensity than levodopa to cause side-effects and they are tolerated less well especially by elderly patients and those with dementia. The ergot derivatives have been associated with pericardial, pleural and retroperitoneal fibrosis.

Direct comparison studies of the different dopamine agonists are lacking but a number of meta-analyses and comparisons of the literature suggest that they have similar efficacy. Individual variations in response and tolerance usually determine which agonist will be used in a particular patient.

Anticholinergics

Anticholinergics have been used in Parkinson's disease for more than 100 years. They have modest antiparkinsonian efficacy and they can be used as initial therapy in mild disease especially when tremor is a main feature. They are relatively ineffective for the more disabling features of PD, such as bradykinesia and rigidity. Anticholinergic agents currently available in the UK are biperiden, procyclidine, orphenadrine, benzhexol and benztropine. Benzhexol and orphenadrine are the most commonly used. Due to a peripheral parasympathomimetic action, side-effects such as dryness of the mouth, blurred vision, urinary retention (especially in those with prostatic hypertrophy), precipitation of closed-angle glaucoma and constipation can occur. Central side-effects include confusion, hallucinations and transient cognitive impairment. Anticholinergics should therefore be used very cautiously in the elderly; they may also be associated with withdrawal effects.

Selegiline

Selegiline is a monoamine oxidase B (MAO-B) inhibitor. MAO-B is one of the enzymes involved in the metabolism of dopamine. Selegiline selectively and irreversibly inhibits intracellular and extracellular MAO-B and therefore reduces or delays the breakdown of dopamine to dihydroxyphenylacetic acid (DOPAC) and hydrogen peroxide. The latter has been implicated in oxidative damage of dopaminergic neurones in the substantia nigra; its possible neuroprotective properties have already been discussed. Selegiline was first introduced as an adjuvant treatment in later disease and added to levodopa it can reduce motor fluctuations.[51] Subsequent studies assessed its efficacy in early disease. In the DATATOP study selegiline delayed the need for levodopa by nine months, a fact that was put down to a mild symptomatic effect of the drug.[10] Although a UK Parkinson's Disease Research Group trial found increased mortality in patients treated with selegiline,[52] further analysis did not confirm these findings.[53] Because of its amphetamine and methamphetamine metabolites it can cause agitation, confusion and significant sleep disturbance. It can be used as initial therapy for young patients (i.e. <65 years of age) without cognitive impairment in the early stages of the disease. The suggested daily dose is 10 mg.

Amantadine

This antiviral agent has been used in Parkinson's disease for almost 30 years. Several mechanisms have been suggested for its antiparkinsonian action including the release of dopamine from dopaminergic neurones, inhibition of dopamine reuptake, anticholinergic action and NMDA glutamate receptor antagonism. The effects of amantadine on parkinsonian symptoms are modest – when given as monotherapy in early disease it results in mild to moderate improvement in two-thirds of patients.[54] There is a suggestion that the beneficial effects of amantadine may be short lived but there is no good evidence for the development of tolerance.[55] Lately there has been a renewed interest in the use of amantadine, as small trials have shown that it is efficacious for treating dyskinesias. Side-effects are central and peripheral and they include confusion, hallucinations, insomnia, nightmares, livedo reticularis and ankle oedema. The dose usually used is 100 mg b.d. but it may be increased, if well tolerated, to 300 or 400 mg daily.

Recommendations

Although controversial, the recent body of information supports the delay of initiation of levodopa as long as the patient's disability allows. Dopamine agonists are the first choice when symptomatic treatment is needed. Dopamine agonists as monotherapy can provide satisfactory control of parkinsonian symptoms, although inferior to that of levodopa, and they are recommended in the early stages of the disease especially in young onset patients who are more prone to develop motor complications. There is also a possibility that they may slow down the progression of the disease. Levodopa supplementation is advised later in the course of the disease, when symptoms are no longer satisfactorily controlled on dopamine agonist monotherapy. However, starting treatment with levodopa is still preferable under certain circumstances. Elderly patients and patients with dementia, as well as patients with pre-existing comorbidity, e.g. hypotension, are more likely to develop side-effects with dopamine agonists. The severity of the disease may also determine drug choice, as patients with severe disease who are at risk of falling or losing a job will need to be treated with levodopa with no delay. Selegiline, amantadine and anticholinergics have modest antiparkinsonian efficacy and they are not considered as first-line drugs for the treatment of PD. These therapeutic options can provide satisfactory control of symptoms for several years until the patient reaches the complex clinical stage. Treatment initiation strategies are listed in the box below.

Box 1.2   Treatment recommendations in early-stage Parkinson's disease

- None of the currently available drugs has proven neuroprotective efficacy
- Initiate therapy with a dopamine agonist, especially in young patients
- Supplement with levodopa when satisfactory control of symptoms is no longer feasible
- Consider adding a COMT inhibitor to levodopa to extend its half-life
- Rarely consider initiation of therapy with anticholinergics, selegiline or amantadine in young patients with mild symptoms or tremor-dominant disease

Management of Late-stage Disease

The complex stage of the disease is characterized by loss of the smooth response to medication and the emergence of motor fluctuations and dyskinesias. Approximately 75–80% of PD patients will eventually develop motor complications, particularly younger individuals.[56] It is estimated that after five years of treatment with levodopa, 50% of patients will suffer from them, while 100% of patients with onset at less than 40 years of age will have motor complications after six years of treatment. Once established, they can be an important source of disability and extremely difficult to control with medication. Moreover, non-motor symptoms and symptoms that do not respond to dopaminergic treatment further debilitate the patient.

Non-motor symptoms include dementia, psychosis, depression, autonomic dysfunction, dysphagia, severe speech problems, postural instability and freezing.

Paramedical therapies, such as physiotherapy, occupational therapy and speech and language therapy are very important for the management of the late stages of the disease (see Chapter 3 for more detail). The specialist nurse can provide significant support with helping the patient with complex medication regimes, liaise with community services and other members of the multidisciplinary team and offer valuable psychological support.

Management of Motor Complications

Before attempting to treat motor complications, each levodopa cycle needs to be well described to enable one to understand the pattern of the motor phenomena and relate them to high or low dopaminergic stimulation; a symptom diary card kept by the patient or the carer can provide significant help. Motor complications can be divided into two main types: motor fluctuations and dyskinesias. Oscillations in the response to the medication and the mobility status are characteristic of fluctuations, while involuntary movements that could be choreic, choreoathetoid or dystonic characterize dyskinesias.

Motor fluctuations

The 'wearing off' phenomenon – an increasingly shortened benefit period following each dose of levodopa – is usually the earliest type of motor fluctuation to occur. Symptoms deteriorate in a regular and predictable manner two to four hours after a levodopa dose or they are worse early in the morning. 'Wearing off' periods may also manifest with non-motor phenomena such as paraesthesia, pain, anxiety, low mood, tachycardia, sweating and shortness of breath.

Lowering individual doses of levodopa and shortening the dosage interval so that the total daily dosage remains unchanged works well initially. Unfortunately, with time the dosage interval may become inconveniently short.

The controlled-release preparations may be tried to substitute partly or totally the immediate-release levodopa. Because of the reduced bioavailability of the controlled-release levodopa the total dosage has to be increased to obtain satisfactory control of the symptoms by 20–60%. Controlled-release preparations can produce a moderate reduction in 'off' time, at the same time allowing a reduction in the numbers of doses of levodopa, but their effects on dyskinesias are variable with a tendency for these to increase.[57]

The addition or increase in dose of a dopamine agonist is more commonly used in clinical practice to reduce fluctuations by smoothing the dopaminergic stimulation.

> Cabergoline, pergolide, pramipexole and ropinirole have been shown to produce significant reduction in 'off' time.[58–61]

The addition of a dopamine agonist may cause increased dyskinesias. In that case, patients are advised to reduce levodopa doses. Most of the dopamine agonists are effective in alleviating other disabling complications such as restless legs syndrome, sleep fragmentation and early morning akinesia or dystonia.

COMT inhibitors are another class of drugs used in fluctuating patients. As an adjunct to levodopa they can decrease 'off' time, increase 'on' time and reduce the required dosage of levodopa,[62,63] although they can enhance dyskinesias.

Selegiline and amantadine may have a mild efficacy in improving short duration responses[64] and they are used more rarely.

Apart from 'wearing off', '*delayed on*' (prolonged latency from drug intake to turning on) and '*no on*' (total dose failure) can also shorten the duration of response to levodopa. Peripheral pharmacokinetic mechanisms related to the absorption of levodopa are believed to be responsible for delayed response to the drug. These include gastroparesis with delayed gastric emptying and interference of heavy protein meals with the absorption of levodopa; the poor solubility of levodopa also contributes to its erratic absorption. Patients are advised to take levodopa one hour before or one hour after meals with greater protein intake in the evening. Crushing the tablets to powder and drinking them with large amounts of water provides additional help. The prescription of gastrokinetic agents, such as cisapride and domperidone, may also be beneficial. A highly soluble prodrug of levodopa (levodopa ethylester) is currently being tested and it is expected to reduce the response latency as well as the number of dose failures.[65]

'*On-off phenomenon*' is characterized by sudden, unpredictable shifts between overtreated states, usually with dyskinesias, and undertreated states with marked akinesia and disability.

Medical management is difficult and patients are often considered for surgery. Initially, the increase of dopaminergic therapy by increasing the dose of levodopa or dopamine agonist, or by adding a COMT inhibitor, may be tried. Unfortunately these interventions will often enhance dyskinesias. Dietary protein manipulation may be effective in smoothing the response to levodopa. In patients with severe fluctuations, changing to liquid levodopa may allow a more reliable and consistent response although this option requires highly motivated patients because of the inconvenience of its very frequent dosing and daily preparation. Subcutaneous apomorphine injections can be used as 'rescue' therapy at intolerable 'off' states but the duration of the effect is short (approximately one hour) and domperidone has to be taken prior to the injection to prevent nausea. Continuous subcutaneous apomorphine infusion is also effective in smoothing symptom control but the cost, the complicated technique that necessitates support by experienced staff and the frequent side-effects limit its use. When none of the available medical treatments is effective, surgical approaches can then be considered (Table 1.1).

Table 1.1 Management of motor fluctuations

Fluctuation	Treatment
'Wearing off'	More frequent dosing of levodopa Add a dopamine agonist or increase its dose Add a COMT inhibitor Substitute partly or totally immediate-release levodopa for controlled-release preparations
'Delayed on' … and dose failures	Restrict protein ingestion; avoid taking levodopa with meals Gastrokinetis (cizapride; domperidone)
'On-off' fluctuations	Increase dopaminergic therapy Add a COMT inhibitor Dietary protein manipulation Apomorphine intermittent or continuous administration Liquid levodopa Surgery

Dyskinesias

There are different subtypes of dyskinesias depending on their relation to the cycle of the doses of levodopa. *'Peak dose'* dyskinesias appear at the peak levodopa concentration and dopaminergic stimulation; they are usually choreic or rarely dystonic. *'Biphasic'* or *'beginning and end of dose'* dyskinesias appear in the intervals when levodopa levels rise and fall, usually in the form of repetitive, stereotyped movements of the lower limbs. *'Off period'* dyskinesias are characterized by dystonic postures of the feet and usually occur early in the morning.

The management of 'peak dose' dyskinesias requires the reduction of individual doses of levodopa, e.g. by 25 mg increments. If this results in exacerbation of the parkinsonian signs a dopamine agonist should be introduced or its dose increased. It is usually easier to manage dyskinetic patients if they are switched from controlled-release to immediate-release levodopa. If a COMT inhibitor has been recently added, a 20–30% reduction in the levodopa dose is usually beneficial.

'Biphasic' dyskinesias are more refractory to management. The patient might benefit from higher doses of the dopaminergic agents. Amantadine is the only agent which has been shown to have anti-dyskinetic effects possibly by inhibiting the overactivity of down-stream glutamatergic pathways. Small trials have reported a reduction in dyskinesias that was often significant.[66,67]

The management of 'off period' dystonia consists mainly of reducing the 'off' time. Specifically for the treatment of trouble-some early morning dystonia, a long-acting dopamine agonist, e.g. cabergoline, or a dose of controlled-release levodopa can be tried at bedtime. Baclofen, anticholinergics and lithium can also be helpful for 'off dystonia' but at the expense of side-effects. Another therapeutic consideration is local injection with botulinum toxin.

In refractory and disabling dyskinesias liquid levodopa, a duodenal levodopa infusion system, a subcutaneous apomorphine pump or surgery may be considered, as shown in Box 1.3.

Management of Non-motor Symptoms

Non-motor symptoms include dementia, neuropsychiatric manifestations, depression, sleep disorders, autonomic dysfunction and

---

Box 1.3   Management of dyskinesias

- Reduce individual doses of levodopa
- Add a dopamine agonist or increase its dose if mobility is compromised
- Add amantadine
- Apomorphine continuous infusion
- Liquid levodopa
- Surgery

---

freezing. The pharmacological aspects of the neuropsychiatric symptoms of Parkinson's disease are described in this chapter; Chapter 2 describes the psychosocial impact and management of the psychiatric features in more detail.

Dementia

A third of PD patients will eventually develop dementia, especially those with an older age at onset.[68] The use of cholinesterase inhibitors in demented PD patients still remains investigational. A study with rivastigmine showed improvement in cognitive function in dementia with Lewy bodies.[69]. Demented patients are much more likely to develop psychiatric side-effects with antiparkinsonian drugs.

Hallucinations and psychosis

Psychiatric adverse events are more likely to occur in patients with dementia, advanced age, premorbid psychiatric illness and exposure to high doses of levodopa. They may be precipitated by concurrent infections, metabolic imbalance or cerebrovascular events. The spectrum of psychiatric side-effects includes visual hallucinations, paranoid delusions, confusion and delirium. They comprise a significant risk factor for nursing home placement and subsequent mortality,[70] hence effective management is of paramount importance.

The first step is to identify and treat a possible precipitating cause. If symptoms are persistent, antiparkinsonian drugs should be gradually discontinued, preferably in the following order: anticholinergics; selegiline; amantadine; dopamine agonists; and COMT inhibitors. If psychosis persists, levodopa dosage should be tapered down to the minimum that permits mobility. If all of these measures are not helpful, or if medication reduction results in significant disability, then atypical neuroleptics can be tried. The most successful of these is clozapine, which, in small doses, provides satisfactory control of PD psychosis without motor compromise.[70] Unfortunately its use is limited by the close monitoring required because of the risk of leucopaenia. Quetiapine is another promising candidate drug to treat psychosis without worsening of parkinsonism.[72] Another approach to the treatment of behavioural problems is the use of cholinesterase inhibitors, which have been shown to improve neuropsychiatric symptoms as well as cognition.[73]

Depression

Depression affects approximately 20% of patients with PD. Patients respond to the use of conventional antidepressants. Sedative antidepressants are preferable for patients with sleep disorders, while stimulating antidepressants are beneficial when apathy predominates. Postural hypotension may prevent the use of tricyclic antidepressants in elderly patients. The combination of an anticholinergic with a tricyclic antidepressant may result in intolerable antimuscarinic side-effects.

Sleep disorders

Sleep fragmentation, vivid dreaming, REM sleep behaviour disorders, excessive daytime sleepiness and altered sleep–wake cycles may interfere with the quality of sleep and therefore directly affect daytime functioning. Sleep fragmentation, probably caused by nocturnal dystonia or increased akinesia, can be ameliorated by a dopamine agonist or controlled-release levodopa given at bedtime, and reducing dopaminergic medication before bedtime can diminish vivid dreaming. Clonazepam is effective for REM sleep behaviour disorders and modafinil, a new stimulant marketed for use in narcolepsy, is helpful in reducing daytime sleepiness.[74]

Autonomic dysfunction

Special attention should be paid to autonomic symptoms as these cause major discomfort to patients. They include postural hypotension, urinary frequency and urgency, impotence, swallowing problems and constipation. Where a non-pharmacological approach is feasible, drugs should therefore be avoided. In cases of severe symptomatic postural hypotension, midodrine (an alpha-1 agonist) or fludrocortisone, can be tried. Tolterodine or oxybutynin can be used to treat bladder dysfunction. Sildenafil can be used to treat erectile dysfunction. Constipation can be managed with dietary modification (increased fluid and fibre intake), increased physical activity, discontinuation of offending drugs (anticholinergics) and the use of mild laxatives. Patients with swallowing problems should be referred to a speech and swallowing therapist.

Postural instability and freezing

When freezing is unrelated to the cycle of levodopa dosage, it is refractory to any kind of treatment. Botulinum toxin injections have been tried with variable effects.[75] Physiotherapy can provide advice on cues to help freezing, and can also be effective in treating postural instability.

Conclusions

Parkinson's disease is a chronic, progressive disorder that can result in severe functional disability and compromise of the quality of life. Medical treatment offers satisfactory control of the symptoms for several years, until the emergence of the long-term complications of dopaminergic therapy that include fluctuations and dyskinesias. Motor complications as well as non-motor symptoms, which appear later in the course of the disease, are difficult to manage and they cause significant distress both to the patient and the carer.

> Both in the early and later stages of PD, optimal management demands both careful pharmacological supervision and a multidisciplinary therapeutic approach.

Multidisciplinary management and approaches to service delivery are discussed in detail in Chapters 3 and 4.

References

1. Goldman SM, Tanner C (1998) Etiology of Parkinson's disease. In: Jankovic J, Tolosa E, eds. *Parkinson's Disease and Movement Disorders*, 3rd ed, 133–58. Lippincott Williams & Wilkins, Baltimore.
2. Mouradian MM (2002) Recent advances in the genetics and pathogenesis of Parkinson's disease. *Neurology* **58**: 179–85.

3. MacMahon DG, Thomas S (1998) Practical approach to quality of life in Parkinson's disease: the nurse's role. *J Neurol* **245** (Suppl. 1): S19–S22.

4. Koller WC (2002) Treatment of early Parkinson's disease. *Neurology* **58**: S79–S86.

5. Tintner R, Jankovic J (2002) Treatment options for Parkinson's disease. *Curr Opin Neurol* **15**: 467–76.

6. Jenner P, Olanow CW (1998) Understanding cell death in Parkinson's disease. *Ann Neurol* **44** (Suppl. 1): S72–S84.

7. Rascol O, Goetz C, Koller W *et al.* (2002) Treatment interventions for Parkinson's disease: an evidence-based assessment. *Lancet* **359**: 1589–98.

8. Shults CW, Oakes D, Kieburtz K *et al.* (2002) Effects of coenzyme Q10 in early Parkinson's disease: evidence of slowing of the functional decline. *Arch Neurol* **59**: 1541–50.

9. Parkinson Study Group (1989) Effects of deprenyl on the progression of disability in early Parkinson's disease. *N Engl J Med* **321**: 1364–71.

10. Parkinson Study Group (1993) Effects of tocopherol and deprenyl on the progression of disability in early Parkinson's disease. *N Engl J Med* **328**: 176–83.

11. Le WD, Jankovic J (2001) Are dopamine receptor agonists neuroprotective in Parkinson's disease? *Drugs Aging* **18**: 389–96.

12. Olanow WC (2002) The role of dopamine agonists in the treatment of early Parkinson's disease. *Neurology* **58**: S33–S41.

13. Marek K, Seibyl J, Shoulson I *et al.* (2002) Dopamine transporter brain imaging to assess the effects of pramipexole vs levodopa on Parkinson's disease: a four-year randomised controlled trial. *Neurology* **58**: A81–A82.

14. Whone A, Remy P, Davis M *et al.* (2002) The REAL-PET study: slower progression in early Parkinson's disease treated with ropinirole compared to L-dopa. *Neurology* **58**: A82–A83.

15. Bhatia K, Brooks DJ, Burn DJ *et al.* (2001) Updated guidelines for the management of Parkinson's disease. *Hosp Med* **62**: 456–70.

16. Lang AE, Lozano AM (1998) Medical progress: Parkinson's disease. *N Engl J Med* **339**: 1130–43.

17. Cotzias GC, van Woert MH, Schiffer LM (1967) Aromatic amino acids and modification of parkinsonism. *N Engl J Med* **276**: 374–9.

18. Koller WC, Hubble JP (1990) Levodopa therapy in Parkinson's disease. *Neurology* **40**: 40–7.

19. Uitti RJ, Ahlskog JG, Maraganore DM, *et al.* (1993) Levodopa therapy and survival in idiopathic Parkinson's disease: Olmsted County Project. *Neurology* **43**: 1918–26.

20. Marsden CD, Parkes JD (1973) On-off effects in patients with Parkinson's disease on chronic levodopa therapy. *Lancet* **1**: 292–6.

21. Filion M (2000) Physiologic basis of dyskinesia. *Ann Neurol* **47**: S35–S40.

22. Brotchie JM (2000) The neuronal mechanism underlying levodopa-induced dyskinesias in Parkinson's disease. *Ann Neurol* **47** (Suppl.): S193–S202.

23. Damier P, Trembay L, Feger J, Hirsch EC (2000) Development of dysk-inesias induced by treatment for Parkinson's disease: potential role of first exposure to L-dopa (or phenomenon of priming). *Rev Neurol (Paris)* **156**: 224–35.

24. Katzenschlager R, Lees A (2002) Treatment of Parkinson's disease: lev-odopa as the first choice. *J Neurol* **249** (Suppl. 2): II/19–II/24.

25. Onofrj M, Paci C, Thomas A (1998) Sudden appearance of invalidating dyskinesia–dystonia and off fluctuations after the introduction of lev-odopa in two dopaminomimetic drug naïve patients with stage IV Parkinson's disease. *J Neurol Neurosurg Psychiatry* **65**: 605–6.

26. Di Monte DA, McCormac A, Petzinger G *et al.* (2000) Relationship among nigrostriatal denervation, parkinsonism and dyskinesias in the MPTP primate model. *Mov Disord* **15**: 459–66.

27. Colzi A, Turner K, Lees AJ (1998) Continuous subcutaneous waking day apomorphine in the long-term treatment of levodopa induced interdose dyskinesias in Parkinson's disease. *J Neurol Neurosurg Psychiatry* **64**: 573–6.

28. Quinn N, Marsden CD, Parkes JD (1982) Complicated response fluctu-ations in Parkinson's disease: response to intravenous infusion of lev-odopa. *Lancet* **21**: 412–15.

29. Poewe WH, Lees AJ, Stern GM (1986) Low-dose L-dopa therapy in Parkinson's disease: a 6-year follow-up study. *Neurology* **36**: 1528–30.

30. Block G, Liss C, Scott R *et al.* (1997) Comparison of immediate-release and controlled-release carbidopa/levodopa in Parkinson's disease: a multicentre 5-year study. *Eur Neurol* **37**: 23–7.

31. Spencer JP, Jenner A, Aruoma OL *et al.* (1994) Intense oxidative DNA damage promoted by L-dopa and its metabolites: implications for neu-rodegenerative diseases. *FEBS Lett* **353**: 246–50.

32. Agid Y (1998) Levodopa. Is toxicity a myth? *Neurology* **50**: 858–63.

33. Quinn N, Parkes D, Janota I, Marsden CD (1986) Preservation of the substantia nigra anad locus coeruleus in a patient receiving levodopa (2 kg) plus decarboxylase inhibitor over a four-year period. *Mov Disord* **1**: 65–8.

34. Lyytinen J, Kaakkola S, Teräväinen H *et al.* (1997) Comparison between the effects of L-dopa + entacapone and L-dopa + placebo on exercise capacity, haemodynamics and autonomic function in patients with Parkinson's disease (abstract). *Mov Disord* **12** (Suppl. 1): 103.

35. Chase TN, Engber TM, Mouradian MM (1996) Contribution of dopa-minergic and glutamatergic mechanisms to the pathogenesis of motor response complications in Parkinson's disease. *Adv Neurol* **69**: 497–501.

36. Nohria V, Partiot A (1997) A review of the efficacy of the dopamine agonists pergolide and bromocriptine in the treatment of Parkinson's disease. *Eur J Neurol* **4**: 537–43.

37. Quinn N (1995) Drug treatment of Parkinson's disease. *BMJ* **310**: 575–9.

38. Shannon KM, Bennett JP Jr, Friedman JH (1997) Efficacy of pramipexole, a novel dopamine agonist, as monotherapy in mild to moderate Parkinson's disease. The Pramipexole Study Group. *Neurology* **49**: 724–8.

39. Adler CH, Sethi KD, Hauser RA *et al.* (1997) Ropinirole for the treatment of early Parkinson's disease. The Ropinirole Study Group. *Neurology* **49**: 393–9.

40. Barone P, Bravi D, Bernejo-Pareja F *et al.* (1999) Pergolide monotherapy in the treatment of early PD: a randomized controlled study. Pergolide Monotherapy Study Group. *Neurology* **53**: 573–9.

41. Lees AJ, Katzenschlager R, Head J, Ben-Shlomo Y, on behalf of the Parkinson's Disease Research Group of the United Kingdom (2001) Ten-year follow-up of three different initial treatments in de-novo PD. *Neurology* **57**: 1687–94.

42. Rascol O, Brooks DJ, Korczyn AD *et al.* (2000) A five-year study of the incidence of dyskinesia in patients with early Parkinson's disease who were treated with ropinirole or levodopa. 056 Study Group. *N Engl J Med* **342**: 1484–91.

43. Rinne UK (1987) Brief communications: early combination of bromocriptine and levodopa in the treatment of Parkinson's disease: a 5-year follow-up. *Neurology* **37**: 826–8.

44. Parkinson Study Group (2000) Pramipexole vs levodopa as initial treatment for Parkinson's disease. *JAMA* **284**: 1931–8.

45. Rinne UK, Bracco F, Chouza C *et al.* (1998) Early treatment of Parkinson's disease with cabergoline delays the onset of motor complications. Results of a double-blind levodopa controlled trial. The PKDS009 Study Group. *Drugs* **55** (Suppl. 1): 23–30.

46. Oertel WH (2000) Pergolide vs levodopa (PELMOPET). *Mov Disord* 15 (Suppl. 3): M86. Data presented at the 6th International Congress of Parkinson's Disease and Movement Disorders (Barcelona, June 11–15, 2000).

47. Stocchi F, Vacca L, De Pandis MF, *et al.* (2001) Subcutaneous continuous apomorphine infusion in fluctuating patients with Parkinson's disease: long-term results. *Neurol Sci* **22**: 93–94.

48. Ondo W, Hunter C, Almaguer M *et al.* (1999) Efficacy and tolerability of a novel sublingual apomorphine preparation in patients with fluctuating Parkinson's disease. *Clin Neuropharmacol* **22**: 1–4.

49. Manson AJ, Hanagasi H, Turner K *et al.* (2001) Intravenous apomorphine therapy in Parkinson's disease: clinical and pharmacokinetic observations. *Brain* **124**: 331–40.

50. Bianchine J, Poole K, Woltering F (2002) Efficacy and dose response of the novel transdermally applied dopamine agonist Rotigotine CDS in early Parkinson's disease. *Neurology* **58**: A162–A163.

51. Oertel WH, Quinn NP (1996) Parkinsonism. In: Brandt T, Caplan LR, Dichgans J *et al.*, eds. *Neurological Disorders. Course and treatment*, 715–72. Academic Press, San Diego.

52. Lees AJ (1995) Comparison of therapeutic effects and mortality data of levodopa combined with selegiline in patients with early, mild Parkinson's disease. Research Group of the United Kingdom. *BMJ* **311**: 1602–7.

53. Ben-Shlomo Y, Churchyard A, Head J *et al.* (1998) Investigation by Parkinson's Disease Research Group of United Kingdom into excess mortality seen with combined levodopa and selegiline treatment in patients with early, mild Parkinson's disease: further results of randomised trial and confidential inquiry. *BMJ* **316**: 1911–16.

54. Butzer JF, Silver DE, Sans AL (1975) Amantadine in Parkinson's disease: a double-blind, placebo-controlled, crossover study with long-term follow-up. *Neurology* **25**: 603–6.

55. Factor SA, Molho ES (1999) Transient benefit of amantadine in Parkinson's disease: The facts about the myth. *Mov Disord* **14**: 515–17.

56. Schrag A, Quinn NP (2000) Dyskinesias and motor fluctuations in Parkinson's disease. A community-based study. *Brain.* **123**: 2297–305.

57. Goetz CG, Tanner CM, Shannon KM *et al.* (1988) Controlled-release long-acting levodopa/carbidopa combination in Parkinson's disease patients with and without motor fluctuations. *Neurology* **38**: 1143–5.

58. Poewe W (1998) Adjuncts to levodopa therapy: dopamine agonists. *Neurology* **50** (Suppl. 6): S23–S26.

59. Lieberman A, Olanow CW, Sethi K *et al.* (1998) A multicenter trial of ropinirole as adjunct treatment for Parkinson's disease. Parkinson Study Group. *Neurology* **49**: 1060–5.

60. Marsden CD (1998) Clinical experience with cabergoline in patients with advanced Parkinson's disease treated with levodopa. *Drugs* **50**: 17–22.

61. Lieberman A, Ranhosky A, Korts D (1997) Clinical evaluation of pramipexole in advanced Parkinson's disease: results of a double-blind, placebo-controlled, parallel-group study. *Neurology* **49**: 162–8.

62. Adler CH, Singer C, O'Brien C *et al.* (1998) Randomized, placebo-controlled study of tolcapone in patients with fluctuating Parkinson's disease treated with levodopa-carbidopa. *Arch Neurol* **55**: 1089–95.

63. Rinne UK, Larsen JP, Siden A, Worm-Petersen J (1998) Entacapone enhances the response to levodopa in parkinsonian patients with motor fluctuations. *Neurology* **51**: 1309–14.

64. Savery F (1977) Amantadine and a fixed combination of levodopa and carbidopa in the treatment of Parkinson's disease. *Dis Nerv Syst* **38**: 605–8.

65. Djaldetti R, Inzelberg R, Giladi N *et al.* (2002) Oral solution of levodopa ethylester for treatment of response fluctuations in patients with advanced Parkinson's disease. *Mov Disord* **17**: 297–302.

66. Verhagen Metman L, Del Dotto P, LePoole K *et al.* (1999) Amantadine for levodopa-induced dyskinesias: a 1-year follow-up study. *Arch Neurol* **56**: 1383–6.

67. Snow BJ, MacDonald L, Mcauley D, Wallis W (2000) The effect of amantadine on levodopa-induced dyskinesias in Pakinson's disease: a double-blind, placebo-controlled study. *Clin Neuropharmacol* **23**: 82–5.

68. Mayeux R, Denaro J, Hemenegildo N *et al.* (1992) A population-based investigation of Parkinson's disease with and without dementia: relationship to age and gender. *Arch Neurol* **49**: 492–7.

69. McKeith I, Del Ser T, Spano P *et al.* (2000) Efficacy of rivastigmine in dementia with Lewy bodies: a randomised, double-blind, placebo-controlled international study. *Lancet* **356**: 2031–6.

70. Goetz CG, Stebbins GT (1993) Risk factors for nursing home placement in advanced Parkinson's disease. *Neurology* **43**: 2227–9.

71. Parkinson Study Group (1990) Low-dose clozapine for the treatment of drug-induced psychosis in Parkinson's disease. *N Engl J Med* **340**: 757–63.

72. Fernandez HH, Friedman JH, Jacques C, Rosenfeld M (1999) Quetiapine for the treatment of drug-induced psychosis in Parkinson's disease. *Mov Disord* **14**: 484–7.

73. Reading PJ, Luce AK, McKeith IG (2001) Rivastigmine in the treatment of parkinsonian psychosis and cognitive impairment: preliminary findings from an open trial. *Mov Disord* **16**: 1171–4.

74. Hauser RA, Wahba MN, Zesiewicz TA, Anderson WM (2000) Modafinil treatment of pramipexole-associated somnolence. *Mov Disord* **15**: 1269–71.

75. Giladi N, Gurevich T, Shabtai H *et al.* (2001) The effect of botulinum toxin injections to the calf muscles on freezing of gait in parkinsonism: a pilot study. *J Neurol* **248**: 572–6.

2

The Psychosocial Impact of Parkinson's Disease and its Clinical Management

Marjan Jahanshahi

Introduction

In this chapter, the aim is to outline the major effects of Parkinson's disease (PD) on the patients and their families in terms of daily life, emotional well-being and healthcare use. The chapter establishes a framework within which the psychosocial impact of PD is best considered and then focuses on the impact of PD on the patient, with the greatest consideration given to depression for two reasons: because it is relatively common in PD and, when present, depression influences the patient's quality of life. The chapter ends with consideration of the various approaches available for management of the psychosocial consequences of PD.

The Stress of Chronic Illness

The diagnosis of PD is experienced as stressful because it is both unexpected and uncontrollable.[1,2] In addition PD is a chronic and progressive illness, hence daily activities and social and occupational functioning show a gradual decline and over time, familiar personal, occupational and social roles may have to be given up and future expectations and aspirations revised. These changes can create a sense of emotional loss which may be associated with the four stages of grieving: feelings of shock and denial, followed by anger, then mourning and depression and finally acceptance.

People differ in how they accept and adjust to a chronic illness such as PD. Dakof and Mendelsohn (1989) described four patterns of adjustment to the illness: sanguine and engaged; depressed and apprehensive; depressed and misunderstood; and passive and resigned.[3] The four groups showing these differing patterns of adjustment were distinguished in terms of presence/absence and severity of depression as well as disease severity but not demographic and health variables. The 'sanguine and engaged' subgroup had the least severe PD and appeared well adjusted. In contrast, the 'depressed and apprehensive' subgroup was characterized by an unsuccessful struggle to cope with the illness and anxiety about the future. The 'depressed and misunderstood' group was the most severely disabled, depressed and socially isolated, and showed a marked withdrawal from participation in previous personal, family and social roles. In comparison, the 'passive and resigned' subgroup had accepted and resigned themselves to their dependence on their carers for self-care and daily activities.

The rate of progress of PD is a major determinant of the psychosocial effects of the illness.[4–6] Coping with a chronic illness such as PD is not a 'one-off' challenge but a continuous and ongoing process of adjustment.[6] The challenges posed by chronic illness change with the phase of illness. For example, in the early phase shortly after diagnosis, when the symptoms are relatively mild, patients have to adjust to the diagnosis, and alter their future plans and expectations. Later, patients enter the 'complex' phase of the disease and develop moderately severe symptoms and disability, as a result of which key social and occupational roles may have to be given up. The late 'palliative' phase of the illness is characterized by severe symptoms that are no longer controlled by medical treatment leading to loss of autonomy and increasing dependence. Emotionally, this phase may be associated with feelings of helplessness as the disease 'takes over' and physical dependence increases.

Research has established that a number of factors influence how well people adjust to and cope with chronic illness.[7–12] The most important of these factors are summarized in Table 2.1 and include illness-related factors such as rate of progression, personal characteristics of individuals such as their sense of self-esteem, their life circumstances such as marital status or financial security,

Table 2.1 Some of the main factors that influence adjustment to and coping with chronic illness

Factor	Parameter
Illness related	Duration of illness
	Rate of progression
	Age of onset
	Controllability of symptoms
Personal characteristics	Gender
	Age
	Beliefs about control
	Appraisal of illness
	Self-esteem
	Self-efficacy
	Coping styles/strategies
Life circumstances	Marital status
	Nature of work
	Financial situation
Social or environmental	Type and suitability of accommodation
	Living alone or with others
	Social support

and the physical and social environment in which the person lives. The impact of PD is therefore determined by a complex interaction between the characteristics of the illness, the person and the environment in which they live.

Disability in Daily Activities

The symptoms of PD result in loss of normal motor function and disability in daily activities. The symptoms of PD are wide ranging and their impact on the patients' or families' daily lives and their social consequences may differ. For example, postural instability and gait problems interfere with mobility whereas hypophonia and masked facies interfere with verbal and non-verbal communication. A number of studies have focused on describing the social impact of PD on patients' daily lives.[13,14] Singer (1973) reported that patients with PD were less likely to work, to have a circle of friends, and do household duties, and were more likely to engage in stationary and solitary activities such as watching television and reading, a pattern considered to reflect 'premature social ageing' in their sample of younger patients.[14] There is evidence that disability, as measured by the Schwab and England scale,[15] is greater in PD patients who had experienced falls than those who had not.[16] Bloem *et al.* (2003) found fear of falling to be common in PD; it was reported by 46% of the 59 patients studied, and led to restriction of activities and, in some cases, social isolation.[17]

Depression

Minor depression is a common experience in PD. Estimates of the prevalence of major depressive illness range from 2.7% to 3.6%[18,19] in community-based samples applying strict diagnostic criteria, to 20%[20] to 90%.[21] Many methodological and sampling factors are likely to contribute to this variability of rates, including the instrument used for diagnosis.[22] Several studies have examined a range of psychiatric symptoms in PD and have found depression to be the most frequently encountered disorder.[23,24]

Characteristics of depression in Parkinson's disease

There is some overlap in the symptoms of PD and depression.

> Bradykinesia in PD and psychomotor retardation in depression, fatigue and apathy in PD and loss of energy and lack of motivation in depression are some of the symptoms common to the two disorders.

The qualitative characteristics of the depression experienced by patients with PD has been described by Gotham *et al.* (1986).[25] Pessimism and hopelessness, decreased motivation and drive, and increased concern with health were the main features of depression in PD, while negative feelings of guilt, self-blame and worthlessness were absent. This pattern was confirmed by Huber *et al.* (1990).[26] These qualitative characteristics of depression in PD relative to the core symptoms of primary depressive illness are also borne out by the low suicide rate in PD – the rate of suicide in the general population in the UK (0.8%) is ten times higher than the rate (0.08%) found in PD.[27]

Changes in depression in Parkinson's disease over time

Since PD is a chronic and progressive disorder, the impact of the illness on daily activities and psychosocial functioning is likely to change over time. A number of studies have examined how disability and depression change with progression of the illness. Mayeux *et al.* (1988) followed 49 PD patients over an average period of 2.5 years.[28] Fourteen of these patients had major depression and seven had dysthymia. Remission occurred in one of the patients with major depression and three with dysthymia; there were no new cases of depression. In a longitudinal follow-up study of 132 patients over a two-year period, Brown *et al.* (1988) found that while mean levels of depression were unchanged, individual patients showed changes in depression.[29] Both baseline and follow-up levels of depression were significantly related to levels of disability. The relative level and rate of increase in disability across time were considered better predictors of depression than its absolute level. In their longitudinal follow-up of a sample of 92 patients with PD for a period of 12 months, Starkstein *et al.* (1992) found that those with major depression at the time of initial assessment showed a significantly greater deterioration in activities of daily living,[30] further progression of illness as indexed by the Hoehn and Yahr scale,[31] and greater cognitive decline than patients with minor depression or no depression.

Association of depression with other features of Parkinson's disease

A previous history of depression, female gender, and greater left-brain involvement have been identified as risk factors for depression in PD in some studies but not others (see Cummings, 1992,[32] for review). A few studies report significant but modest associations between depression and duration and severity of PD[30,33] while others found no such association.[34–37] Celesia and Wanamaker (1972) found that depression was most common in Hoehn and Yahr[31] stages I (38%), III (42%) and IV (50%) but less frequent in stages II (18%) and V (22%).[36] This pattern was replicated by Starkstein *et al.* (1990) who also found that depression was high in stage I (around the time of disease onset/diagnosis), fell in stage II (perhaps when patients come to accept the reality of the diagnosis, and levodopa successfully controls the symptoms of PD), increased in stages III and IV (coincidentally with progression of the illness and development of drug-induced complications) and fell again in stage V (when patients perhaps become resigned to their dependency on others).[37] This triphasic and non-linear association shows that in PD the association between depression and disease processes is complex.

In contrast, depression in PD has been associated with several other features of the disorder, particularly cognitive impairment and age of onset. Mayeux *et al.* (1981) first noted a modest but significant association between severity of depression and cognitive impairment in PD when assessing 55 non-demented patients with PD.[33] Starkstein *et al.* (1989) assessed a consecutive series of 105 patients and found that the 15 PD patients with major depression performed significantly worse on a battery of tests of cognitive function, particularly those assessing 'frontal' executive function, than an age and stage of illness-matched subgroup of 15 patients with no depression.[35] Starkstein *et al.* (1990, 1992) found cognitive decline over a follow-up period of 3–4 years (1990 study) or one year (1992 study) to be significantly greater for those PD patients who were depressed at the time of baseline assessment than non-depressed patients.[30,37] The PD patients with major depression also showed significantly faster progression of PD and deterioration of activities of daily living than those with minor or no depression.

Age of onset of PD is another factor that has been shown to influence depression in PD, with patients with early-onset PD (onset before age 55) being significantly more depressed than patients with late-onset PD, even after controlling for differences in the duration of illness.[39,40] In the late-onset group, depression significantly correlated with impairments in activities of daily living, while in the early-onset group, cognitive impairment and duration of illness were the main correlates of depression.[40]

Recently, Schrag *et al.* assessed psychosocial function in 75 patients with onset of PD before the age of 50, and 66 patients with later onset in greater detail.[41] Other than a higher rate of drug-induced motor complications, the young- and old-onset groups did not differ in disease severity or disability. The young-onset group had higher rates of unemployment due to disability, lower marital satisfaction, higher divorce rates, lower levels of satisfaction with emotional and mental support, worse quality of life (as measured by the PDQ-39) and higher rates of moderate-to-severe depression on the Beck Depression Inventory (40% vs 17%) than the old-onset group. The coping strategies used by two groups also differed: the young-onset patients used 'acting out' and 'distraction' strategies more frequently than older-onset patients who used 'distancing' strategies more often.

'On-off' fluctuations are among the complications of long-term levodopa therapy. There is evidence that these fluctuations in motor function, where the patient shifts from being mobile (on) to being akinetic (off) may also be accompanied by alterations of mood and cognition at least in some cases. Several investigators have reported mood swings with greater depression or anxiety/panic in the 'off' state.[42–46] In a sample of 136 PD patients studied by Nissenbam *et al.* (1987), 23% had 'on-off' fluctuations, 69% of whom experienced greater depression in the 'off' state.[45] For the majority of the ten patients studied by Menza *et al.* (1990) mood improved significantly from the 'off' to the 'on' state but then deteriorated in the 'on with dyskinesia' state, which suggests that besides changes in dopamine levels, the functional disability experienced by the patients in the 'off' or 'on with dyskinesia' state also plays a part in these alterations of mood.[44]

Predictors of depression in Parkinson's disease

As shown in Table 2.1, the personal characteristics, life circumstances of individuals, and the physical and social environment all affect a patient's ability to participate in family life and society. Brown and Jahanshahi (1995) suggested a model of the major factors contributing to depression in PD. This model shown in Figure 2.1, is multivariate and considers both biological and psychological influences on depression in PD.[47]

Therefore, it is proposed that a complex web of disease-related processes and interrelated social and personal factors operate to determine a patient's coping and adjustment to chronic illnesses such as PD. The contribution of illness-related and psychosocial factors to depression in PD has been empirically examined in a number of studies. To date, the study by MacCarthy and Brown (1989) has been the most comprehensive investigation of the psychosocial determinants of depression and adjustment of illness in PD.[8] They examined the association between disability, self-esteem, attributions and perceived control, social support, coping strategies and depression and adjustment to illness in 136 patients

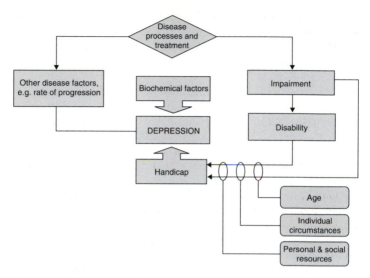

Figure 2.1   Brown and Jahanshahi's (1995) model for the major factors producing or influencing depression in Parkinson's disease.[47]

with PD. Disability in activities of daily living, self-esteem and use of maladaptive coping strategies such as wishful thinking or denial accounted for 44% of the variance of depression in PD. Disability and the use of maladaptive coping strategies were also major predictors of adjustment of illness, and availability of practical social support contributed to positive well-being in this sample.

Anxiety and Other Psychiatric Features

Many symptoms of PD can give rise to anxiety. The unpredictability of function associated with 'on-off' fluctuations, the disturbance of posture and balance, and the risk of falls when walking are among the symptoms likely to contribute to anxiety. Since these symptoms of PD are perceived as making mobility around the house and outside prone to falls they can give rise to 'fear of falling', which as noted above is quite common in PD, reported by 46% of patients.[17] Because of this fear of falling, mobility – particularly venturing outside the home – can be considered as risky and is therefore often avoided. This avoidance can ultimately result in social isolation.

While depression in PD has been directly and extensively studied, specific research on anxiety in PD is more limited. Stein *et al.* (1990) studied 24 patients with PD and found that 9 (38%) had anxiety disorder according to DSMIII-R criteria.[48] The severity of anxiety was not correlated with severity of PD symptoms, duration or dose of levodopa therapy. Other studies have also found anxiety to be a common experience in patients with PD.[24,25,49] The comorbidity of anxiety and depression in PD has been reported in a number of studies.[50,51] Among the 99 patients assessed on the Beck Depression Inventory, Beck Anxiety Scale and the Fatigue Severity Scale, Shulman *et al.* (2001) found that 36% reported depression, 33% anxiety and 40% fatigue.[51]

Other psychiatric symptoms such as hallucinations, delusions, fatigue and apathy are also features of PD, each of which can have an impact on the patient's daily activities and quality of life. Hallucinations are common symptoms, reported by 26% of 102 consecutive patients.[52]

Fatigue is one of the symptoms of PD which is likely to contribute to disability. Krupp and Pollina (1996) defined fatigue as 'an overwhelming sense of tiredness, lack of energy and feeling of exhaustion'.[53] Fatigue may be physical, mental or emotional. Although fatigue is among the symptoms of depression, many *non-depressed* PD patients also report significant fatigue.[54–56] For example, van Hilten *et al.* (1993) found that 43% of non-depressed patients with PD reported fatigue.[55] One-third of PD patients rated fatigue as their most disabling symptom and more than 50% considered fatigue as among their three most disabling symptoms; this tends to be persistent.[54,57] The relation between fatigue and disease severity and anti-parkinsonian medication is inconsistent across studies.[55,56] Despite the fact that fatigue is reported as a disabling symptom by a large proportion of PD patients, to date its contribution to the quality of life of patients has not been investigated.

Apathy consists of reduced motivation and lack of affect. The percentage of patients with PD who experience apathy in the absence of depression varies from 5%[58] to 17%.[24] As with fatigue, apathy can also contribute to disability and poor quality of life in PD but so far these associations have not been directly investigated.

Quality of Life

The term 'health-related QoL' encompasses the sum total effect of the illness and its medical treatment on an individual's physical, psychological, social and occupational functioning as perceived by that individual. Comprehensive management of a person with chronic illness aims to promote a good quality of life for the affected person, their primary carer and their family.

QoL measures are now considered better indices of the impact of chronic illness than measures of impairment or disability. Both disease-specific and generic measures of QoL have been used in PD and are discussed in Chapter 5.

Depression has emerged as a major predictor of QoL in PD across a number of studies.[59,60] In a population-based study, Schrag et al. set out to identify the demographic and disease-related determinants of QoL in PD.[61–63] They used the PDQ-39[64] a disease-specific QoL measure, and two generic measures, the SF36 and the EURO-Qol.[65] Using regression analysis, Schrag et al. established that depression, disability, postural instability and cognitive impairment were the predictors of QoL in PD, accounting for 72% of the variance of QoL scores.[63] The 124 PD patients had a poorer QoL compared to the general population of the same age, particularly in the domains of physical mobility and social functioning.[61]

Stage of illness and age of onset have also been identified as important determinants of QoL in PD.[59–61,66,67] In 86 PD patients, Koplas et al. (1999) obtained ratings of QoL on a single 5 point Likert scale.[67] They found that while disability and depression increased with stage of illness, QoL and perceived mastery over life decreased. In a more recent study, Schrag et al. directly compared 75 young-onset (onset before 50) and 66 older-onset PD patients.[41] They found that QoL measured on the PDQ–39 was significantly worse for the young-onset group, with perceived stigmatization, lack of social support, impaired cognition, reduced emotional well-being, disability in activities of daily living, impairment of mobility and communication skills all being significantly higher for the young-onset than the old-onset patients.

Perceived Stigma

The symptoms of PD such as rigidity and tremor, and drug-induced dyskinesias, are evident to other people and can make the sufferer appear 'different' – this can result in stigmatization. Stigma is a concept with a social dimension and relates to the interaction of the patient with his wider social milieu. Goffman (1963) originally defined stigma in terms of any condition, behaviour, trait or attribute that in some way marked the person as 'different', 'culturally or socially unacceptable' or 'inferior'.[68] In their study, Schrag *et al.* examined perceived stigma in patients with young-onset versus old onset PD[41]; perceived stigma was significantly higher for the patients with young-onset PD than for those with old-onset disease. This difference is interesting. The slowness, rigidity and mobility problems of PD are perhaps to a lesser extent features of the normal ageing process and in this sense probably less stigmatizing when they occur in elderly PD sufferers than in younger patients who would be expected to be fit and healthy. Drug-induced dyskinesias which tend to develop early and be more severe in patients with young-onset PD,[69] may also contribute to the higher perceived stigma in these patients.

Other Effects of Parkinson's Disease

Impact of Parkinson's disease on the carer and family

The family operates as a 'system' in which the state of health and daily functioning of individual members affects their interactions with the other members and has implications for their collective functioning and well-being.[70] When one member falls ill, the functioning of the whole system is affected and its previously balanced working may be disturbed. To compensate for this, individual members, such as the spouse and children, may have to alter their behaviour and take on new roles. Thus, PD affects the whole family, not just the ill person. The illness has major implications for the present and future life of the spouse and children, particularly those who may still be living at home.[6]

Children

To date, only two studies have examined the impact of PD on children. Grimshaw (1991) interviewed young children of PD sufferers and found that most children were aware of parental disease, particularly adolescents who were somewhat embarrassed by it, but that this had no negative impact on school performance or friendships.[71] Some families expressed a need for specific help in relation to children. Schrag *et al.* developed a scale for assessing the impact of parental illness on adolescent and adult children.[72] Using this Impact of Parental Illness Scale (IPIS), 99 subjects aged between 19 and 48 who had a parent with PD were assessed. Parental PD had a marked impact on the well-being of their adolescent or *adult children* as measured on the IPIS. Impact of parental PD increased with longer disease duration. Younger children still living in the parental home reported a higher burden of daily help and greater impact on their social interactions. Mild to moderate depression was reported by one-fifth of the children.

Carers

In the last few years, the impact of PD on the spouse has been assessed in a number of studies. O'Reilly *et al.* (1996) compared the physical, psychological and social functioning of spouses of PD patients who did or did not act as carers for their ill spouse.[73] They found that spouses who acted as carers were significantly less likely to get out of the house at least once a week than the spouses who were not carers and that contact with friends and neighbours decreased with increasing care provision. The psychological health scores of the spouses who were carers were significantly worse and these carers had a five-fold increase in psychiatric morbidity. Thus caring for their spouse with PD affected their physical, psychological and social well-being.

Subsequent studies have examined the factors that contribute to the caregiving strain experienced by the spouse. Carter *et al.* (1998) examined the influence of stage of illness on the experiences of 380 caregivers, all of whom were the patients' spouses.[74] While caregiver physical health and preparedness for their caregiving role did not differ across the five stages of illness, caregiver depression was significantly higher by stages IV and V. Mutuality (i.e. the extent to which the caregivers enjoyed their time with their spouse who had PD) declined from stage II. From stage 2.5, caregiving spouses reported significant negative lifestyle changes. Of 51 possible caregiving activities, the mean number carried out by the spouses was 11 at stage I but this increased to an average of 30 at stages IV and V. Early in the course of the illness, the spouses received almost no help from others, but help from relatives, friends or paid helpers increased significantly in the later stages of PD (stages IV and V). As expected from these results, caregiver strain was experienced across all five stages but became significantly greater as PD progressed.

In a small cohort of 45 patients with PD and their spouses, Fernandez *et al.* (2001) examined what contributed to depression in the spouses of PD patients.[75] The depression scores of the spouses showed a moderate but significant association ($r = 0.35$, $p = 0.02$) with the severity of PD symptoms rated on the UPDRS, age of onset ($r = 0.33$, $p = 0.02$), duration ($r = 0.43$, $p = 0.003$) and depression scores of the PD patients ($r = 0.29$, $p < 0.05$). While spouse depression was significantly higher for those PD patients with sleep disturbance than those without, the presence of hallucinations, delusions, cognitive impairment or incontinence in the PD patient had no significant effect on spouse depression. In stepwise regression analysis, PD duration of illness emerged as the only significant predictor of the variance of spouse depression scores in this study. In contrast, an earlier study by Aarsland *et al.* (1999) found that mental symptoms in PD patients, such as depression, severity of psychiatric symptoms (delusion; agitation; aberrant motor behaviour) and cognitive impairment, were the predictors of depression and emotional distress in the spouses.[24] Miller *et al.* (1996) also found that depression in PD patients was a major contributor to depression in the caregiver but that the availability of social support did not predict carer distress.[76] Overall, these findings suggest that the presence of cognitive deficits and psychiatric symptoms such as depression and delusions in the PD patient contribute more towards the emotional distress experienced by the primary carers than do other factors such as social support.

Impact of Parkinson's disease on healthcare use

Parkinson's disease, which has a mean disease duration of about 15 years, has major implications for healthcare use. In the UK, in 1992, it was estimated that the NHS spent £383 million each year on the care of people with PD.[77] The cost of medication and compensation for lost earnings are among the most significant expenses. Evidence also shows that this cost is greater for PD patients with dyskinesias and 'on-off' fluctuations than those without.[78,79] The health burdens of PD increase with the progression of the illness and are greater in the advanced than early stages.[77,79] Both direct (e.g. community services; modification of home/car; use of aids and equipment) and indirect (e.g. early retirement/ unemployment) health economic indices were found to be significantly affected by stage of illness[66] and were greater for more advanced disease.

There is also evidence that in PD, as in other chronic disorders,[80,81] the patient's healthcare use is not solely determined by illness-related parameters but that psychosocial factors such as depression and social support are important in this respect.[82] De Boer *et al.* (1999) found that during a 6 months period, the average number of consultations with a neurologist or GP were respectively 1.9 and 1.1.[82] In addition, 48% of the 235 patients had seen a physiotherapist and 20% had a home care nurse as compared to only 8% having seen a psychotherapist during the same period. While the predictors of neurologist visits were availability of private health insurance and living with others, GP visits were predicted by poorer social functioning and QoL. Lack of social support and poor QoL as well as disease duration and severity were predictors of use of physiotherapy, home care nurses and psychotherapy. Thus, psychosocial factors such as QoL influence the patient's use of medical (GP visits) and non-medical care.

Clinical Management of the Psychosocial Consequences of Parkinson's Disease

Improvement of the symptoms of PD through medical treatment will reduce their impact on daily activities and is likely to be of value in the management of the psychosocial sequel of the illness. However, as the sole course of action, such a medical approach is unlikely to be completely effective for preventing disability and depression and promoting good QoL in PD for several reasons:

- Some symptoms, such as postural instability, gait problems, and cognitive impairment are not very responsive to levodopa.[16,17,83]
- The relationship between impairment, activity and participation is non-linear.[47]
- A multitude of person-related, social and environmental factors operate to influence an individual's adjustment to PD.
- As noted above, healthcare use is influenced by factors such poor social support.

How is the psychosocial impact of PD best managed? Various approaches may prove of value. These include direct drug therapy for depression and anxiety, informing and educating the patient, and provision of cognitive-behavioural therapy.

Drug therapy for depression

The overlap between the symptoms of PD and the symptoms of depression and anxiety may make it difficult for the neurologist to identify depression and anxiety in PD patients. The masked facies, low voice, lack of affect and apathy that may characterize some PD patients may also make it less likely for them to successfully communicate feelings of depression or anxiety to the neurologist. However, evidence suggests that neurologists do reliably identify depression and other mood disorders during routine consultations.[84] Given that depression and anxiety are common in PD and likely to change in the course of the illness, the neurologist and GP need to enquire about these from the patient and carer at every consultation.

When present, major depression and anxiety in PD need direct treatment. The efficacy of tricyclic antidepressants for treatment of depression in PD has been established in double-blind trials,[85] although these may produce more side-effects in PD than selective serotonin reuptake inhibitors (SSRIs). The latter class of drugs has not been subjected to double-blind trials in PD, although in a survey of specialists, SSRIs were the treatment of choice for depression in PD,[86] and open-label case studies have shown SSRIs such as sertraline to be effective in treating depression in PD.[87] However, as noted by a recent report of the Task Force of the Movement Disorders Society (2002), there is currently insufficient evidence from controlled studies about the value of SSRIs for treatment of depression in PD.[88]

Informing and educating the patient

The provision of information about PD, its medical treatment and its likely course may be helpful to the patient in two important ways. First, it will, at least to some extent, prepare patients and their families for what to expect in the coming years. Second, it may allow them to recruit the personal, social and financial resources that may be essential for coping with the impact of the illness on their daily activities, work and social relationships. In turn, this would promote a greater sense of personal control and overcome feelings of helplessness.

Educating patients about a number of general principles is also likely to help them cope better with their motor disability. Examples of such general principles are as follows:[6,89]

- breaking down complex actions into a number of steps and then performing them one step at a time

- ensuring that they do not do two things at once but perform tasks one at a time
- timing activities to coincide with periods of maximum mobility
- allowing plenty of time for travelling or completion of tasks
- paying attention to each movement as they perform them.

PD group exercise and education sessions improve patient and carer understanding of the disease and its treatment and are a useful means of conveying and re-enforcing the principals that underpin PD rehabilitation and management strategies. The only controlled study to examine the value of an educational pro-gramme is by Montgomery et al. (1994) who found that while activities of daily living remained stable in the 'intervention' group provided with PD-specific educational material, it showed further deterioration in the 'control' group.[90] This information helps patients realize the range of potential interventions and can improve patients' communication with healthcare professionals. Encouraging patients to recruit a network of relatives and friends who can provide them, their carers and families with emotional and practical support at times of need may be of value.[11,91] Frequent, open and honest communication with the carer and children about any problems associated with PD may help promote better interaction between family members. The role of adjunct therapies and nurse specialists in maintaining functioning and quality of life is discussed in Chapters 3 and 4 respectively.

Cognitive-behavioural therapy

As outlined above, depression and anxiety are quite common in PD but they can both be successfully treated with cognitive-behav-ioural techniques.[92,93] First, the patient needs to accept that they have PD, accept its limitations, adjust to the restrictions imposed by it and set themselves realistic goals and standards, e.g. by allow-ing more time for daily tasks. This is important in preventing dis-appointment and self-blame if previous standards are not achieved. Second, patients have to appreciate that their thoughts, feelings and behaviour are closely related, and learn to monitor their thoughts to establish how what they think affects the way they feel and behave. The negative thinking style characteristic of depres-sion means that the depressed individuals perceive themselves, the world and the future in negative terms.[92,93] Similarly, the thought processes of the anxious individual are marked by a sense of threat and danger. With training, depressed and anxious patients can learn to identify and challenge negative thoughts and the errors of thinking which result in biased interpretations of reality. Relaxation training for counteracting any physical symptoms of anxiety and arousal, which can act to magnify anxiety or fear, would also be of value. Where severe avoidance and restriction of activity have developed (e.g. due to fear of falling) systematic desensitization or 'graded exposure' to the feared situations may be necessary. To protect their sense of self-esteem, patients need to realize that despite the physical changes produced by the illness, their past achievements have not been altered and that there are no obstacles to reaching new and realistic goals. Given that psychosocial factors also contribute to the development of depression in PD (see Figure 2.1) patients should also be encouraged to remain active and not to give up professional or social roles prematurely. New activities and hobbies can be pleasurable in the short-term and also help promote a sense of control and achievement. Given the importance of practical and emotional social support in protecting individuals emotionally against the effects of the stress of chronic illness,[11,91] patients should maintain their social ties with friends and family.

A programme of training in coping skills incorporating stress inoculation, positive thinking, social skills training, modelling and role play, and muscle relaxation was used by Ellgring et al. (1998) to teach 25 patients with PD to accept the reality of their illness, cope with being in public places and deal with difficult situations.[49] Although the value of the programme delivered as five two-hour seminars in the course of two months was not systematically assessed, it was rated as very helpful by the patients. To date, the only controlled study of the efficacy of behavioural therapy for PD has been that of Muller et al. (1997) who compared 15 patients randomly assigned to behavioural intervention with 14 receiving non-specific psychological and physical therapy.[94] The behavioural intervention programme included a combination of education (e.g. breaking down complex movements to simple components), positive reinforcement and relaxation training; this lasted ten weeks with two 90-minute sessions per week. At follow-up, significant improvement on the Hoehn and Yahr, UPDRS motor and ADL scores were observed for the patients in the intervention group. While the results of these studies are positive, as concluded by the Task Force of the Movement Disorders Society (2002), there is insufficient evidence about the value of psychosocial intervention in PD.[95] Further well-designed studies are clearly required.

Conclusions

Parkinson's disease has a major psychological and social impact on patients, their carers and their children and has implications for healthcare use. A range of approaches for successful clinical management of the psychosocial consequences are available, which can help patients and their families adjust to and live well with PD.

References

1. Paykel ES (1997) The interview for recent life events. *Psychol Med* **27**(2): 301–10.
2. Paykel ES, Cooper Z, Ramana R, Hayhurst H (1996) Life events, social support and marital relationships in the outcome of severe depression. *Psychol Med* **26**(1): 121–33.
3. Dakof GA, Mendelsohn GA (1989) Patterns of adaptation to Parkinson's disease. *Health Psychol* **8**: 355–72.
4. Mindham RH, Bagshaw A, James SA, Swannell AJ (1981) Factors associated with the appearance of psychiatric symptoms in rheumatoid arthritis. *J Psychosom Res* **25**: 429–35.
5. Moos RH, Solomon GF (1965) Personality correlates of the degree of functional incapacity of patients with physical disease. *J Chronic Dis* **18**: 1019–38.
6. Jahanshahi M, Marsden CD (1998) *Living and coping with Parkinson's disease: A self-help guide for patients and their carers.* Human Horizon Series, Souvenir Press, London: 337.
7. Felton BJ, Revenson TA (1984) Coping with chronic illness: a study of illness controllability and the influence of coping strategies on psychological adjustment. *J Consulting Clin Psychol* **52**: 343–53.
8. MacCarthy B, Brown R (1989) Psychosocial factors in Parkinson's disease. *Br J Clin Psychol* **28**: 41–52.
9. Jahanshahi M, Marsden CD (1990) Body concept, disability and depression in torticollis. *Behav Neurol* **3**: 117–31.
10. Jahanshahi M, Marsden CD (1990) A longitudinal follow-up study of depression, disability and body concept in torticollis. *Behav Neurol* **3**: 233–46.
11. Jahanshahi M (1991) Psychosocial correlates of depression in torticollis. *J Psychosomatic Res* **35**: 1–15.
12. Folkman S, Lazarus RS (1985) If it changes it must be a process: study of emotion and coping during three stages of a college examination. *J Pers Soc Psychol* **48**: 150–70.

13. Oxtoby M (1982) *Parkinson's disease patients and their social needs.* Parkinson's Disease Society, London.

14. Singer E (1973) Social costs of Parkinson's disease. *J Chron Dis* **26**: 243–254.

15. Schwab RS, England AC (1969) Projection technique for evaluating surgery in Parkinson's disease. In: Gillingham FJ, Donaldson IML, eds, *Third Symposium on Parkinson's disease.* E & S Livingstone, Edinburgh: 152–157.

16. Koller WC, Glatt S, Vetere-Overfield B, Hassanein R (1989) Falls and Parkinson's disease. *Clin Neuropharmacol* **12**(2): 98–105.

17. Bloem BR, Grimbergen YAM, Cramer MC *et al.* (2003) Prospective assessment of falls in Parkinson's disease. *J Neurol* (in press).

18. Hantz P, Caradoc-Davies G, Caradoc-Davies T, Weatherall M, Dixon G. Depression in Parkinson's disease. *Am J Psychiatry* 1994; **151**(7): 1010–14.

19. Tandberg E, Larsen JP, Aarsland D, Cummings JL (1996) The occurrence of depression in Parkinson's disease. A community-based study. *Arch Neurol* **53**(2): 175–9.

20. Patrick HT, Levy DM (1992) Parkinson's disease: a clinical study of 146 cases. *Arch Neurol Psychiatry* **7**: 711–20.

21. Mindham RH (1970) Psychiatric syndromes in Parkinsonism. *J Neurol Neurosurg Psychiatry* **30**: 188–91.

22. Slaughter JR, Slaughter KA, Nichols D *et al.* (2001) Prevalence, clinical manifestations, etiology, and treatment of depression in Parkinson's disease. *J Neuropsychiatry Clin Neurosci* **13**(2): 187–96.

23. Brown RG, MacCarthy B (1990) Psychiatric morbidity in patients with Parkinson's disease. *Psychol Med* **20**(1): 77–87.

24. Aarsland D, Larsen JP, Lim NG *et al.* Range of neuropsychiatric disturbances in patients with Parkinson's disease. *J Neurol Neurosurg Psychiatry* **67**: 492–6.

25. Gotham AM, Brown RG, Marsden CD (1986) Depression in Parkinson's disease: a quantitative and qualitative analysis. *J Neurol Neurosurg Psychiatry* **49**(4): 381–9.

26. Huber SJ, Friedenberg DL, Paulson GW *et al.* (1990) The pattern of depressive symptoms varies with progression of Parkinson's disease. *J Neurol Neurosurg Psychiatry* **53**: 275–8.

27. Myslobodsky M, Lalonde F, Hicks L (2001) Are patients with Parkinson's disease suicidal? *J Geriatr Psychiatry Neurol* **14**: 120–4.

28. Mayeux R, Stern Y, Sano M *et al.* (1988) The relationship of serotonin to depression in Parkinson's disease. *Mov Disord* **3**(3): 237–44.

29. Brown RG, MacCarthy B, Gotham AM, *et al.* (1988) Depression and disability in Parkinson's disease: a follow-up of 132 cases. *Psychol Med* **18**(1): 49–55.

30. Starkstein SE, Mayberg HS, Leiguarda R *et al.* (1992) A prospective longitudinal study of depression, cognitive decline, and physical

impairments in patients with Parkinson's disease. *J Neurol Neurosurg Psychiatry* **55**: 377–82.

31. Hoehn MM, Yahr MD (1967) Parkinsonism: onset, progression and mortality. *Neurology* **17**: 427–42.

32. Cummings JL (1992) Depression and Parkinson's disease: a review. *Am J Psychiatry* **149**(4): 443–54.

33. Mayeux R, Stern Y, Rosen J, Leventhal J (1981) Depression, intellectual impairment, and Parkinson's disease. *Neurology* **31**(6): 645–50.

34. Gotham AM, Brown RG, Marsden CD. Depression in Parkinson's disease: a quantitative and qualitative analysis. *J Neurol Neurosurg Psychiatry* 1986; **49**(4): 381–9.

35. Ehmann TS, Beninger RJ, Gawel MJ, Riopelle RJ (1990) Depressive symptoms in Parkinson's disease: a comparison with disabled control subjects. *J Geriatr Psychiatry Neurol* **3**(1): 3–9.

36. Celesia GG, Wanamaker WM (1972) Psychiatric disturbances in Parkinson's disease. *Dis Nerv Syst* **33**: 577–83.

37. Starkstein SE, Bolduc PL, Mayberg HS *et al.* (1990) Cognitive impairments and depression in Parkinson's disease: a follow-up study. *J Neurol Neurosurg Psychiatry* **53**(7): 597–602.

38. Starkstein SE, Bolduc PL, Preziosi TJ, Robinson RG (1989) Cognitive impairments in different stages of Parkinson's disease. *J Neuropsychiatry Clin Neurosci* **1**(3): 243–8.

39. Santamaria J, Tolosa E, Valles A (1986) Parkinson's disease with depression: a possible subgroup of idiopathic parkinsonism. *Neurology* **36**(8): 1130–3.

40. Starkstein SE, Berthier ML, Bolduc PL *et al.* (1989) Depression in patients with early versus late onset of Parkinson's disease. *Neurology* **39**: 1441–5.

41. Schrag A, Hovris A, Morley D *et al.* (2002) Young vs old onset Parkinson's disease: Impact of disease and psychosocial consequences. *Mov Disord* (submitted).

42. Brown RG, Marsden CD, Quinn N, Wyke MA (1984) Alterations in cognitive performance and affect–arousal state during fluctuations in motor function in Parkinson's disease. *J Neurol Neurosurg Psychiatry* **47**(5): 454–65.

43. Cantello R, Gilli M, Riccio A, Bergamasco B (1986) Mood changes associated with 'end-of-dose deterioration' in Parkinson's disease: a controlled study. *J Neurol Neurosurg Psychiatry* **49**(10): 1182–90.

44. Menza MA, Sage J, Marshall E *et al.* (1990) Mood changes and 'on-off' phenomena in Parkinson's disease. *Mov Disord* **5**(2): 148–51.

45. Nissenbaum H, Quinn NP, Brown RG *et al.* (1987) Mood swings associated with the 'on-off' phenomenon in Parkinson's disease. *Psychol Med* **17**(4): 899–904.

46. Raudino F. Non motor off in Parkinson's disease. *Acta Neurol Scand* 2001; **104**(5): 312–15.

47. Brown RG, Jahanshahi M (1995) Depression in Parkinson's disease: A psychosocial viewpoint. In Weiner WJ, Lang AE, eds, *Behavioural Neurology of Movement Disorders*. Advances in Neurology, Volume 65, Raven Press, New York.

48. Stein MB, Heuser IJ, Juncos JL, Uhde TW (1990) Anxiety disorders in patients with Parkinson's disease. *Am J Psychiatry* **147**(2): 217–20.

49. Ellgring H, Seiler S, Nagel U *et al.* (1998) Psychosocial problems of Parkinson patients: Approaches to assessment and treatment. In: Streifter MH, Korczyn AD, eds, *Advances in Neurology*, Volume 53, Raven Press, New York.

50. Menza MA, Robertson-Hoffman, DE, Bonapace AS (1993) Parkinson's disease and anxiety: comorbidity with depression. *Biol Psychiatry* **34**(7): 465–70.

51. Shulman LM, Taback RL, Bean J, Weiner WJ (2001) Comorbidity of the nonmotor symptoms of Parkinson's disease. *Mov Disord* **16**(3): 507–10.

52. Holroyd S, Currie L, Wooten GF (2001) Prospective study of hallucinations and delusions in Parkinson's disease. *J Neurol Neurosurg Psychiatry* **70**(6): 734–8.

53. Krupp LB, Pollina DA (1996) Mechanisms and management of fatigue in progressive neurological disorders. *Curr Opin Neurol* **9**(6): 456–60.

54. Friedman J, Friedman H (1993) Fatigue in Parkinson's disease. *Neurology* **43**(10): 2016–18.

55. Van Hilten JJ, Weggeman M, van der Velde EA *et al.* (1993) Sleep, excessive daytime sleepiness and fatigue in Parkinson's disease. *J Neural Transm Park Dis Dement Sect* **5**(3): 235–44.

56. Karlsen K, Larsen JP, Tandberg E, Jorgensen K (1999) Fatigue in patients with Parkinson's disease. *Mov Disord* **14**(2): 237–41.

57. Friedman JH, Friedman H. Fatigue in Parkinson's disease: a nine-year follow-up. *Mov Disord* 2001; **16**(6): 1120–2.

58. Levy ML, Cummings JL, Fairbanks LA *et al.* (1998) Apathy is not depression. *J Neuropsychiatry Clin Neurosci* **10**(3): 314–9.

59. Kuopio AM, Marttila RJ, Helenius H *et al.* (2000) The quality of life in Parkinson's disease. *Mov Disord* **15**(2): 216–23.

60. Global Parkinson's Disease Survey Steering Committee (2002) Factors impacting on quality of life in Parkinson's disease. Results from an international survey. *Mov Disord* **17**: 60–67.

61. Schrag A, Jahanshahi M, Quinn N (2000) How does Parkinson's disease affect quality of life? A comparison with quality of life in the general population. *Mov Disord* **15**: 1112–18.

62. Schrag A, Selai C, Jahanshahi M, Quinn NP (2000) The EQ-5D – a generic quality of life measure – is a useful instrument to measure quality of life in patients with Parkinson's disease. *J Neurol Neurosurg Psychiatry* **69**: 67–73.

63. Schrag A, Jahanshahi M, Quinn NP (2000) What contributes to quality of life in patients with Parkinson's disease? *J Neurol Neurosurg Psychiatry* **69**: 308–12.

64. Peto V, Jenkinson C, Fitzpatrick R, Greenhall R (1995) The development and validation of a short measure of functioning and well-being for individuals with Parkinson's disease. *Qual Life Res* **4**: 241–8.

65. EuroQoL Group (1990) EuroQoL: a new facility for the measurement of health-related quality of life. *Health Policy* **16**: 199–208.

66. Chrisclilles EA, Rubenstein LM, Voelker MD *et al.* The health burdens of Parkinson's disease. *Mov Disord* **13**: 406–13.

67. Koplas PA, Gans HB, Wisely MP *et al.* (1999) Quality of life and Parkinson's disease. *J Gerontol A Biol Sci Med Sci* **54**(4): M197–M202.

68. Goffman E (1963) *Stigma: Notes on the management of spoiled identity.* Penguin, London.

69. Kostic V, Przedborski S, Flaster E, Sternic N (1991) Early development of levodopa-induced dyskinesias and response fluctuations in young-onset Parkinson's disease. *Neurology* **41**: 202–5.

70. Minuchin S (1974) *Families and Family Therapy.* Harvard University Press, Cambridge, MA.

71. Grimshaw R (1991) *Children of parents with Parkinson's disease. A research report for the Parkinson's Disease Society* National Children's Bureau (NCP) Publications, London.

72. Schrag A, Morley D, Quinn N, Jahanshahi M (2002) Impact of parental Parkinson's disease on adolescent and adult children: The parental illness impact scale (Parkinson's disease). *Psychol Med* (submitted).

73. O'Reilly F, Finnan F, Allwright S *et al.* (1996) The effects of caring for a spouse with Parkinson's disease on social, psychological and physical well-being. *Br J Gen Pract* **46**(410): 507–12.

74. Carter JH, Stewart BJ, Archbold PG *et al.* (1998) Living with a person who has Parkinson's disease: the spouse's perspective by stage of disease. Parkinson's Study Group. *Mov Disord* **13**(1): 20–8.

75. Fernandez HH, Tabamo RE, David RR, Friedman JH (2001) Predictors of depressive symptoms among spouse caregivers in Parkinson's disease. *Mov Disord* **16**(6): 1123–5.

76. Miller E, Berrios GE, Politynska BE. Caring for someone with Parkinson's disease: Factors that contribute to distress. *Int J Geriatr Psychiatry* 1996; **11**(3): 263–8.

77. Dodel RC, Eggert KM, Singer MS *et al.* (1998) Costs of drug treatment in Parkinson's disease. *Mov Disord* **13**(2): 249–54.

78. Dodel RC, Berger K, Oertel WH (2001) Health-related quality of life and healthcare utilisation in patients with Parkinson's disease: impact of motor fluctuations and dyskinesias. *Pharmacoeconomics* **19**(10): 1013–38.

79. Maurel F, Lilliu H, Le-Pen C (2001) [Social and economic cost of L-dopa-induced dyskinesias in patients with Parkinson's disease.] *Rev Neurol* **157**(5): 507–14. French.

80. Traver GA (1988) Measures of symptoms and life quality to predict emergent use of institutional health care resources in chronic obstructive airways disease. *Heart Lung* **17**(6 Pt 1): 689–97.

81. Cronan TA, Shaw WS, Gallagher RA, Weisman M (1995) Predicting health care use among older osteoarthritis patients in an HMO. *Arthritis Care Res* **8**(2): 66–72.

82. De Boer AG, Sprangers MA, Speelman HD, de Haes HC (1999) Predictors of health care use in patients with Parkinson's disease: a longitudinal study. *Mov Disord* **14**(5): 772–9.

83. Bloem BR, van Vugt JPP, Beckley DJ (2001) Postural instability and falls in Parkinson's disease *Adv Neurol* **87**: 209–23.

84. Bridges KW, Goldberg DP (1984) Psychiatric illness in inpatients with neurological disorders: patients' views on discussion of emotional problems with neurologists. *BMJ* **289**: 656–8.

85. Klaassen T, Verhey FR, Sneijders GH *et al.* (1995) Treatment of depression in Parkinson's disease: a meta-analysis. *J Neuropsychiatry Clin Neurosci* **7**(3): 281–6.

86. Richard IH, Kurlan R (1997) A survey of antidepressant drug use in Parkinson's disease. Parkinson Study Group. *Neurology* **49**(4): 1168–70.

87. Hauser RA, Zesiewicz TA (1997) Sertraline for the treatment of depression in Parkinson's disease. *Mov Disord* **12**(5): 756–9.

88. Task Force of the Movement Disorders Society (2002) Treatment of depression in idiopathic Parkinson's disease. *Mov Disord* **17** (Suppl. 4): 112–19.

89. Morris M, Iansek R, Kirkwood B (1995) *Moving Ahead with Parkinson's Disease.* Kingston Centre, Victoria, Australia.

90. Montgomery EB Jr, Lieberman A, Singh G, Fries JF. Patient education and health promotion can be effective in Parkinson's disease: a randomized controlled trial. PROPATH Advisory Board. *Am J Med* 1994; **97**(5): 429–35.

91. Siegal BR, Calsyn RJ, Cuddihee RM (1987) The relationship of social support to psychological adjustment in end-stage renal disease patients. *J Chronic Dis* **40**(4): 337–44.

92. Beck AT (1972) *Depression: Causes and Treatment.* University of Pennsylvania Press, Philadelphia.

93. Beck AT (1976) *Cognitive Therapy and the Emotional Disorders.* New York International Universities Press, New York.

94. Muller V, Mohr B, Rosin R *et al.* (1997) Short-term effects of behavioral treatment on movement initiation and postural control in Parkinson's disease: a controlled clinical study. *Mov Disord* **12**(3): 306–14.

95. Task Force of the Movement Disorders Society (2002) Psychosocial counseling in Parkinson's disease. *Mov Disord* **17** (Suppl. 4): 160–2.

3

Non-pharmacological Therapies

Katherine Deane and Diane Playford

Introduction

The introduction of levodopa therapy in 1967 revolutionized the treatment of Parkinson's disease.[1] Levodopa therapy produces obvious clinical improvement in motor function as tremor, rigidity and bradykinesia respond dramatically to the medication.[2] However, axial signs such as rising from a chair, turning over in bed, posture, gait and postural equilibrium are known to respond less well to levodopa treatment,[3–5] and despite optimal drug management patients develop progressive disability. The development of this disability and the impact it has on patients' roles may be minimized by non-pharmacological therapies. This chapter examines the use of non-pharmacological therapies in Parkinson's disease. We have selected those therapies for which randomized controlled trials in Parkinson's disease have been made. The selection reflects both current paramedical practice within the NHS and the increasing interest in complementary therapies.

What is Rehabilitation?

'Rehabilitation is a process of active change by which a person who has become disabled acquires the knowledge and skills needed for optimum physical, psychological and social function.[6] This definition recognizes that the disabled person plays an active role in determining the end points of the rehabilitation process and how they may be reached.

The aims of rehabilitation will vary between individuals and between client groups. In general the aim is to provide individuals and their families with the knowledge, skills and support necessary to maintain their autonomy, minimize disability and maximize the level of participation of an individual.[7,8] This includes prevention of complications and secondary disability.

At a practical level rehabilitation is a process which consists of a number of stages, which include:

1. Assessment of physiological, psychological and social aspects.
2. Planning of short-term, intermediate or long-term goals.
3. Intervention to help patients achieve these goals.
4. Evaluation of what patients can do at a particular point as compared to the goals previously set.

> Parkinson's disease is chronic and degenerative, therefore interventions that are put in place at one stage may be insufficient or inappropriate at a later stage. Thus the process of rehabilitation in Parkinson's disease is a cyclical one.

Definition of therapies

Therapies are harder to define than drug or surgical interventions. The methods used by therapists are based upon principles but are tailored to the needs of the individual patient. All therapies have a greater or lesser element of education and, in order to gain (maximum) effect, patients are expected to be active participants in their therapeutic programmes. Because of this individual approach it is hard to define precisely what the intervention consists of when looking at a population of patients. However, if the principles and the framework in which they are applied are defined, the disease-specific techniques are described and the level of evidence to support each practice is stated, then a set of evidence-based practice guidelines can be produced. These guidelines can inform therapists in their day-to-day practice and can also be tested within the context of a trial. Such guidelines have been created for physiotherapy[9] and are in development for occupational therapy. Speech and language therapy has general guidelines for the treatment of dysarthria but they are not specific to Parkinson's disease.[10] No specific guidelines exist for Parkinson's disease, for osteopathy, massage therapy or the Alexander Technique.

Principles of therapy

All of the therapies discussed are based upon a number of defined principles (Table 3.1). One principle that is common to them all is that the therapy should be patient centred and tailored to patients' specific needs and ambitions. Another is that patients can be empowered by education and thus enabled to continue the therapeutic process after the intervention by the therapist has been completed. A principle shared with medicine is that prevention is better

Table 3.1 Principles informing therapists in their treatment of people with Parkinson's disease

Therapy	Principles
All	Therapy should be patient centred and tailored to specific needs Patients can be empowered by education and thus enabled to continue the therapy alone Prevention is better than cure The whole is greater than the sum of its parts
Physiotherapy	Physical activity is essential for good health
Occupational therapy	Productive occupation is essential for good health Occupation has physical, psychological and social aspects
Speech and language therapy for dysarthria	Communication is essential for good health
Osteopathy	Structure affects function
Alexander Technique	Voluntary movements can be under conscious and reasoned control 'The relationship of the head to the body in movement is the key to freedom and ease of motion'[58] Excessive and inappropriate muscular activity can be stopped voluntarily (in the absence of illness or injury)
Massage	—

than cure, thus most therapists believe that they should see people with Parkinson's disease early in order to educate them and to stop the development of preventable complications, such as frequent falls, contractures, pressure sores and poor posture.

As often with so many degenerative conditions, the manifestation of a disease is largely dependent on a person's overall well-being and total physical burdens. Therapists tend towards a holistic model of healthcare and this is reflected in techniques that address not only the physical aspects of the disease but also the social and psychological aspects. An activity common to all of these professional groups is counselling. Counselling is 'the means by which one person helps another to clarify their life situation and to decide upon further lines of action.'[11] The care provided also often addresses general health maintenance rather than simply ameliorating the symptoms of the disease (Table 3.2). There is increasing awareness of the importance of self-management, with patients in partnership with clinicians.

Table 3.2   Aims of therapies when treating people with Parkinson's disease

Therapy	Aim
Physiotherapy	To improve or maintain gait, balance, mobility and posture[9]
	To improve or maintain general (cardiovascular) fitness
	To improve or maintain flexibility and range of movement
	To prevent contracture of muscles
Occupational therapy	To improve or maintain functional abilities, independence, safety and confidence
	To remedy occupational deprivation
Speech and language therapy for dysarthria	To improve the intelligibility of speech
	To improve a person's ability to communicate
Osteopathy	To improve structure
Alexander Technique	'A technique by means of which desirable conditions of normality can be restored and maintained'[53]
	To improve ease of motion
	To improve mental discipline
Massage	To improve muscular relaxation

Multidisciplinary therapy

The therapies discussed here are often complementary to one another, as well as to medical and surgical interventions, since they individually work on different components of health and disease, or on similar components in a different way. Therefore they are best placed within a co-operative system of healthcare with efficient teamwork and interprofessional dialogue, so that a balanced set of treatments can be given, generating care that responds to all levels of the person's needs. Despite the consensus amongst paramedical therapists that multidisciplinary working leads to optimum care for patients there are no trials of co-ordinated multidisciplinary input.

The patient is an essential part of the multidisciplinary team. Patients can feel bombarded with many therapists assessing them or coming into their homes, which can lead to confusion and a loss of privacy. A key worker is often essential to balance and co-ordinate care and this person is most commonly the Parkinson's disease nurse specialist.

The aims of each of the therapies are implemented differently according to the principles that inform the therapists. So, for example, although both physiotherapists and occupational therapists may work to improve transfers, they will approach this goal in different ways and with differing overall aims. The physiotherapist aims to increase muscular strength and flexibility with specific exercises, as well as teaching better movement strategies. The overall aim is to enable the patient to get out of the chair, say, as independently as possible. The occupational therapist, on the other hand, will generally assess the height and stability of the chair that the person is transferring from, teach movement, cueing and concentration strategies, and determine why the person needs to get in and out of that chair. The overall aim here is to enable the patient to get out of the chair and so perform the occupation that requires them to be able to transfer. In this context, occupation is the meaningful use of activities, skills and life roles that enable people to function purposefully.[12]

Working to general principles enables therapists in all disciplines to treat a person with Parkinson's disease fairly effectively. The therapists do recognize, however, that Parkinson's disease can lead to some unique difficulties that require disease-specific knowledge, which can often be provided by a Parkinson's disease nurse specialist or the Parkinson's Disease Society.

If therapists had greater access to postgraduate training in disease-specific techniques such as cueing it would undoubtedly improve the general standard of care for people with Parkinson's disease.

Levels of evidence

Consensus used to be informally developed amongst experts in a field as to the most effective therapies and their methods of delivery. In the current climate of evidence-based medicine, opinions, no matter how expert, are insufficient to justify the use of a particular therapy for a disease. Evidence is required so that the size of effect can be estimated more accurately, adverse events can be anticipated or prevented, and the cost of an intervention can be calculated. Randomized controlled trials are not the be all and end all in evidence but they do allow the production of 'bullet-proof' evidence – evidence that is hard to deny and hard to ignore. If well designed, the trial produces evidence that is as free of bias as possible and so can give an objective assessment of the efficacy of a given therapy. A systematic summary of the evidence provides the clinician with a summary of all the evidence in one field, with a clear methodology that can be examined and criticized for possible sources of bias.

However, it should be recognized that randomized controlled trials are only suitable for interventions whose effects are probably moderate in size but clinically worthwhile. Interventions whose efficacy is large and immediately obvious do not require such an examination. For example, a 'chair-raiser' does not need a randomized controlled trial to be proven to be efficacious for people with difficulty in rising from a chair.

Another problem with this form of evidence is its lack of subjective knowledge. One of the great assumptions of trials is that patients are all the same. This is obviously untrue, and so many patients are used to measure the average response to a given therapy. However, in the clinical setting you are dealing with an individual. In the rush to embrace the importance of evidence-based medicine it is easy to lose sight of the knowledge that supports the feelings and intuitions of both patients and therapists. The clinical team should remember that decisions about patient care in a disease such as Parkinson's are always based on insufficient information. It is impossible to predict accurately the responses to a given drug or therapy, as the variables are too great. Therefore subjective knowledge, in the form of clinical judgement, bridges the gap. Subjective knowledge and its inherent flexibility has to be included in care strategies or the patient is likely to feel that their individuality is being ignored.

Criteria for inclusion

In an attempt to provide clinicians with a summary of the objective evidence for non-pharmacological rehabilitation therapies for Parkinson's disease this chapter only examines randomized controlled trials, including, however, trials using quasi-random methods of allocation (such as alternate allocation). We searched an extensive range of electronic databases to locate suitable trials (see Appendix A, p.74), discovering trials for physiotherapy, occupational therapy, speech and language therapy for dysarthria, osteopathy, the Alexander Technique and massage. Other therapies that have been suggested as effective in Parkinson's disease are speech and language therapy for dysphagia, conductive education, acupuncture and chiropractic medicine, but without randomized controlled trials their efficacy, risk and cost cannot be established in the treatment of people with Parkinson's.

Description of the trials

Twenty-five randomized controlled trials examined paramedical and complementary therapies in 750 Parkinson's disease patients. Because the trials had methodological flaws which could have introduced bias, used heterogeneous therapy methods and measured many different outcomes, we could not summarize the results quantitatively by meta-analysis (Tables 3.3, 3.4), so we performed a systematic qualitative appraisal.

Methodological quality of the trials

The trial methods varied in quality (Table 3.5 and Appendix B, p. 76), and all trials had at least one methodological flaw which could have introduced bias. No trial examined had the combination of an adequate method of randomization, adequate concealment of the allocation, blinded assessors and an adequate placebo. These four quality items are generally regarded as having

Table 3.3 Characteristics of studies comparing paramedical therapies with control intervention

Study	Design	Number of patients	Mean baseline Hoehn and Yahr stage*	Total time with therapist (hrs)	Duration of therapy (wks)	Location	Description of therapy	Control intervention
Physiotherapy								
Gibberd 1981[21,22]	Crossover	24	NA	NA	4	Outpatient	Bobath and Peto PNF exercises	Adequate
Hurwitz 1989[14]	Parallel	30	1.6	16	35	Home	National Parkinson's Foundation exercises	Adequate
Cerri 1994[16]	Parallel	6	NA	15	3	Outpatient	Neurofacilitation exercises	None
Comella 1994[18]	Crossover	18	NA	12	4	Outpatient	PNF-based exercises	None
Forkink 1996[19]	Parallel	11	2.7	NA	10	Outpatient	Strengthening of legs, and balance training	None
Katsikitis 1996[24]	Parallel	16	NA	8	4	Outpatient	Orofacial	None
Patti 1996 [19]	Parallel	20	3.4	NA	4	Inpatient	'Rehabilitation'	Inadequate
Thaut 1996[26]	Parallel	22	2.6	10.5	3	Home	Walking exercises	Inadequate

Table 3.3 Continued

Study	Design	Number of patients	Mean baseline Hoehn and Yahr stage*	Total time with therapist (hrs)	Duration of therapy (wks)	Location	Description of therapy	Control intervention
Homann 1998[23]	Parallel	15	2.2	NA	5	Outpatient	Bobath PNF exercises	None
Schenkman 1998[25]	Parallel	51	2.7	30	10–13	Outpatient	Spinal flexibility exercises	None
Chandler 1999[17]	Parallel	67	2.6	NA	52	Home	'Rehabilitation'	Inadequate
Occupational Therapy								
Gauthier 1987[34]	Parallel	64	2.8	20	5	Outpatient	Group OT	Unclear
Fiorani 1997[33]	Parallel	20	NA	12	4	Outpatient	Group OT and physiotherapy	Inadequate
Speech and language therapy								
Robertson 1984[31]	Parallel	22	NA	40	2	Outpatient	Respiration, loudness and prosody	None
Johnson 1990[35]	Parallel	12	NA	10	4	Outpatient	Prosodic exercises	None
Ramig 2001[36]	Parallel	29	2.7	16	4	Outpatient	Increased loudness (LSVT®)	None

Table 3.3 Continued

Study	Design	Number of patients	Mean baseline Hoehn and Yahr stage*	Total time with therapist (hrs)	Duration of therapy (wks)	Location	Description of therapy	Control intervention
Osteopathy								
Wells 1999[46]	Parallel	20	NA	0.75	1	Outpatient	Osteopathic manipulative treatment	Adequate
Alexander Technique and massage								
Stallibrass 2002[47,48]	Parallel	93	NA	16	12	Outpatient	Alexander Technique/lessons or massage	Inadequate

LSVT®, Lee Silverman Voice Therapy®; NA, not available; OT, occupational therapy; PNF, proprioceptive neuromuscular facilitation.

* Although the Hoehn and Yahr scale provides ordinal data most of the authors of the papers provided the mean value.

Table 3.4 Characteristics of studies comparing two forms of paramedical therapies

Study	Design	Number of patients	Mean baseline Hoehn and Yahr stage	Total time with therapist (hrs)	Duration of therapy (wks)	Location	Description of therapy A	Description of therapy B
Physiotherapy								
Palmer 1986[31]	Parallel	14	2.4	36	12	Outpatient	Karate exercises	Standard
Hirsch 1996[28]	Parallel	17	2.0	NA	10	Outpatient	Strength and balance	Balance alone
Muller 1997[29]; Mohr 1996[30]	Parallel	41	2.1	30	10	Outpatient	Behavioural (inc. cues)	Standard
Thaut 1996[26]	Parallel	26	2.5	10.5	3	Home	Walking with auditory cues	Walking without cues
Homann 1998[23]	Parallel	16	NA	NA	5	Outpatient	Bobath	PNF
Shiba 1999[32]	Crossover	8	NA	NA	NA	Outpatient	Walking with visual cues	Walking with auditory cues
Marchese 2000[27]	Parallel	20	2.4	NA	6	Outpatient	Cued	Standard

Table 3.4 Continued

Study	Design	Number of patients	Mean baseline Hoehn and Yahr stage	Total time with therapist (hrs)	Duration of therapy (wks)	Location	Description of therapy A	Description of therapy B
Speech & Language Therapy								
Scott 1983[44,55]	Parallel	64	NA	10	2	Home	Prosodic exercises with visual feedback	Prosodic exercises alone
Ramig 1995, 1996, 1999, 2000;[38-42]; Smith 1995[43]	Parallel	20	2.5	16	4	Outpatient	Increased vocal loudness (LSVT®)	Respiration therapy

LSVT®, Lee Silverman Voice Therapy®, NA, not available, PNF, proprioceptive neuromuscular facilitation.

Table 3.5 Methodological quality of included studies

Quality item	Adequate	Not stated	Inadequate	Total
Randomization method	8	11	6	25
Concealment of allocation	5	13	7	25
Co-interventions constant				
(e.g. drug therapy)	17	7	1	25
Placebo therapy	3	1	14	18
Withdrawals described and				
<10% of original population	15	1	9	25
Blinded assessors	11	11	3	25
Missing values present for				
<10% of original population	15	2	8	25
Intention-to-treat data analysis	9	5	11	25
Between group statistical				
data comparison	17	5	3	25

the greatest impact on the validity of a trial's results. For example, only eight trials truly randomized allocation to treatment groups; of these, only five adequately concealed allocation. Fifteen of the 18 trials with an 'inactive' control arm failed to use a placebo intervention. We defined an adequate placebo therapy intervention as one that provided an inactive 'treatment' to patients for a similar period of time and in a similar setting as the active therapy arm. Eleven of the 25 trials either failed to examine baseline differences or were unbalanced due to small sample sizes. Although the trials examined many outcome measures there was no consensus on which were the most appropriate. Poor presentation and inadequate statistical analysis often hampered interpretation of the results (Tables 3.6, 3.7).

Outcome measures

Many of the trials concentrated on specific physical impairment outcomes such as stride length or vocal loudness but a recent international survey of people with Parkinson's disease found that the physical aspects of the disease accounted for only 17% of the patients' loss of quality of life.[13] It is increasingly recognized that whilst improvement in a specific impairment is easily measured it may have little benefit for the patients in their day-to-day activities.

Table 3.6 Statistically significant results in studies comparing paramedical therapies with control intervention

Outcome	Intervention	Number of studies that measured outcome	Number of studies that calculated statistical significance or provided data in a form that could be analysed	Number of studies with statistically significant results	Calculated P values
Quality of life	Physio	1	0	0	
	OT	1	0	0	
	S&LT	0	0	0	
	Osteo	0	0	0	
	AT	0	0	0	
	Massage	0	0	0	
Speech intelligibility	S&LT	0	0	0	
Activities of daily living	Physio	2	1	1	$P = 0.016$
	OT	2	0	0	
	S&LT	0	0	0	
	Osteo	0	0	0	
	AT	1	1	1	$P = 0.01$
	Massage	1	1	0	
Impairments: summary scores	Physio	3	1	1	$P < 0.01$
	OT	1	0	0	
	S&LT	2	1	1	$P < 0.05$

Table 3.6 Continued

Outcome	Intervention	Number of studies that measured outcome	Number of studies that calculated statistical significance or provided data in a form that could be analysed	Number of studies with statistically significant results	Calculated P values
	S&LT	2	1	1	P < 0.05
	Osteo	0	0	0	
	AT	0	0	0	
	Massage	0	0	0	
Impairments: walking velocity	Physio	5	4	2	P = 0.02; P = 0.01
	OT	1	0	0	
	Osteo	1	1	0	
Impairments: stride length	Physio	3	2	2	P = 0.0045; P = 0.016
	OT	0	0	0	
	Osteo	1	1	1	P < 0.022
Impairments: objective speech loudness	S&LT	2	1	1	P < 0.005

Physio, physiotherapy; OT, occupational therapy; S&LT, speech and language therapy; Osteo, osteopathy; AT, Alexander Technique.

Table 3.7 Summary of the results from studies comparing two forms of paramedical therapy

	Physiotherapy (7 studies)	Speech therapy (2 studies)
Quality of life	Behavioural = Standard[29,30]	LSVT® > Respiration (P not stated)[38–43]
Speech intelligibility	NA	LSVT® > Respiration (carers assessment) (P not stated)[38–43]
		LSVT® = Respiration (patient assessment)[38–43]
Activities of daily living	Strength and balance > balance (P < 0.05)[28]	NA
	Cued = Standard[27]	
	Behavioural = Standard[29,30]	
	Karate = Standard[31]	
Impairments: summary scores	Cued > Standard (P < 0.02)[27]	NA
	Behavioural > Standard (P = 0.01)[29,30]	
Impairments: walking velocity	Walking + auditory cues > walking (P = 0.03)[26]	NA
Impairments: subjective speech loudness	NA	LSVT® = Respiration[38–43]

The authors of the studies defined the statistical significance of data when compared between the two therapy groups.
The '=' refers to no statistically significant difference having been found.
LSVT®, Lee Silverman Voice Therapy®; NA, not appropriate.

Treatment at Different Disease Stages

Diagnosis

People with Parkinson's disease at the diagnosis stage often require no medication and have very little disability. Only one physiotherapy trial examined patients who were at this stage or in the early part of the maintenance stage of the disease (mean Hoehn and Yahr score 1.6). Hurwitz[14] examined the effect of a series of home exercises (15 patients) compared with home visits (15 patients). The author did not provide any raw data, only the results of statistical analysis. Thus the size of any change due to physiotherapy could not be assessed.

No randomized controlled trials examined the efficacy of occupational therapy at this stage of the disease. However, a recent survey of 150 occupational therapists working with people with Parkinson's within the UK showed that 83% of them thought that patients should be referred to an occupational therapist at diagnosis.[15] Dysarthria often occurs later in the disease's progression, so there are few patients who require speech and language therapy at diagnosis, which explains why there were no trials at this stage of the disease. Osteopathy massage and the Alexander Technique aim to improve the general level of health and well-being of the patients. They could all be relevant to patients at diagnosis but no trials were performed at this stage of the disease.

Maintenance

At maintenance, patients are treated with dopaminergic drugs. They usually have a good response to them and few adverse effects. Their level of disability increases as the disease progresses. The majority of trials were performed with patients at this stage of the disease.

Nine trials compared physiotherapy with placebo or no treatment in 230 patients at the maintenance stage of the disease.[16–26] The physiotherapy techniques, duration and location in the trials varied considerably (see Table 3.3). Three trials had interventions from other therapists or had components of their protocol that could be described as occupational therapy.[17,18,21,22] The occupational therapy components were poorly defined and the focus of the trials was mostly on mobility.

A summary of the results is given in Tables 3.6 and 3.7. Only Chandler and Plant[17] measured quality of life but they did not give a full statistical analysis of their results. The trials measured several individual motor impairments but only two outcomes were measured in more than one trial: walking velocity in four trials[17,23,25,26] and stride length in two trials (see Table 3.6).[23,26] Walking velocity increased significantly, in one trial, by 50%[26] but no significant improvement was seen in the other trial.[25] Stride length also improved significantly, in one trial, by 23%.[26] No data for walking velocity or stride length was available in one trial.[23]

Physiotherapy

Seven trials compared two forms of physiotherapy in 142 patients (see Table 3.3).[23,26–32] The majority of outcomes measured were reported to have improved after the 'novel' therapy under investigation (see Table 3.7). One of the techniques used is cueing, which is the prompting of a movement by an external auditory or visual cue such as rhythmic music or lines on the floor, to improve gait. Four of the trials explicitly mentioned the use of cueing in their therapy techniques,[26,27,29,30,32] two of which compared physiotherapy techniques with and without cueing.[26,27] In both of these studies the addition of cueing techniques improved the efficacy of the physiotherapy (see Table 3.7).

Occupational therapy

Two trials examined occupational therapy in 84 patients at this stage of the disease (see Table 3.3).[33,34] These differed markedly in their methodology. Gauthier et al.[34] compared group occupational therapy with an untreated control group whereas Fiorani et al.[33] compared group occupational therapy and physiotherapy with individualized physiotherapy. Fiorani's method of occupational therapy included game playing and basketry as major components of the therapy.[33] Neither trial compared data statistically between groups and therefore it was impossible to determine the statistical significance of differences due to the occupational therapy (see Table 3.6).

Speech and language therapy

Three trials compared speech and language therapy with placebo in 63 parkinsonian patients with dysarthria at this stage of the disease.[35–37] The methods differed considerably (see Table 3.3). No trial measured quality of life, speech intelligibility or activities of daily living affected by poor communication (see Table 3.6). In two trials,[35,36] loudness of speech increased significantly, by 5–12 dB (8–17%) from a mean baseline loudness of 60 dB. Ramig *et al.* showed that this improvement was maintained after six months.[36]

Two trials compared two methods of speech and language therapy in 71 patients.[38–45] Ramig *et al.* and other investigators measured aspects of quality of life affected by speech with the communication subsection of the Sickness Impact Profile.[38–43] The communication subsection score improved by a significant 61% (baseline score of 29) immediately after Lee Silverman Voice Therapy® (LSVT®) as compared to respiration therapy but this improvement was not maintained after 12 months (see Table 3.7). Both trials measured intelligibility on 100-point visual analogue scales but only Ramig *et al.* compared the therapy groups statistically.[38–43] Although patients noticed no difference in outcome between the two therapy modes, their carers found them more intelligible after LSVT®. Ramig *et al.* measured several individual measures of speech quality up to two years after therapy.[42]

Osteopathy

Only one small trial of 20 patients examined the effectiveness of osteopathic manipulation in the treatment of Parkinson's.[46] The study examined the impact of a single treatment session on a number of parameters of gait. The stride length increased significantly by 9%; hip and shoulder velocities also increased significantly by 14%.

Alexander Technique

One trial of 93 patients examined the effectiveness of the 24 Alexander Technique lessons (32 patients) compared to one group treated with therapeutic massage (31 patients) and one untreated group (30 patients).[47,48] Activities of daily living improved in the Alexander group as compared to the untreated group immediately after the intervention; this improvement was still significant six months later. The Alexander group's activities of daily living scores were also significantly better than the massage group after six months, although not immediately after the intervention. Depression scores also improved immediately after Alexander lessons but this improvement was not maintained after six months. Patients in either the untreated control group or the massage group were seven times more likely to change their medication due to worsening symptoms than the Alexander-trained group over the course of the study.

Although the group receiving therapeutic massage improved their activities of daily living immediately after the course of treatment, this improvement was not statistically significant nor was it maintained for six months. None of the other outcomes measured improved significantly in the massage group as compared to the untreated control group.

Complex

At the complex stage of the disease, patients become less responsive to dopaminergic drugs, often needing add-on drugs to smooth 'on and off' periods and often starting to experience dyskinesia. The only study that examined patients with a more complex disease profile was by Patti et al.[49] This was also the only trial that was performed in an inpatient setting. This physiotherapy trial had a poorly defined multidisciplinary component that included occupational therapy. They measured activities of daily living on several scales after intensive inpatient physiotherapy. The four weeks of intensive therapy did result in the greatest number of statistically significant outcomes. All the scales showed improvements that were maintained for five months. Walking velocity increased significantly by 64% and stride length improved significantly by 23%. However, it is questionable how practical it would be to apply this protocol within the current structure of the NHS, and the cost-effectiveness of the intervention was not assessed.

No randomized controlled trials examined the efficacy of any of the other therapies at this stage of the disease.

Palliative

No randomized controlled trials examined the efficacy of any therapy at this stage of the disease. It is probable that this is partly due to the increased practical difficulties of transporting these patients who are often wheelchair bound. Given the degree of co-morbidity and mortality at this stage of the disease, long-term follow-up is problematic.

The lack of physiotherapy trials may also be because there is a perception that such trials have more limited benefit at this stage of the disease due to the patients' severe lack of mobility. It may be more beneficial at this stage to teach carers coping strategies such as lifting and turning techniques.

Nearly all (99%) occupational therapists in a recent survey agreed that occupational therapy is a lifelong need for people with Parkinson's disease.[15] Occupational therapists, particularly those working in social services departments, can provide the larger aids and adaptations that are often required at this stage. They can also support families and ensure that patients remain at home for as long as possible or facilitate transfer to care homes.[50]

Discussion: implications for practice

Because of methodological flaws, the small number of patients examined and the possibility of publication bias, the trials provide insufficient evidence to support or refute the efficacy of these paramedical and complementary therapies in Parkinson's disease. We emphasise that the current lack of evidence for efficacy of these treatments does not imply a lack of effect, rather that further work is required. Large pragmatic randomized controlled trials are needed to assess the effectiveness of paramedical therapies in Parkinson's disease.

Clinically useful recommendations can therefore, at present, only be supported by various levels of subjective knowledge. We have given our opinions, supported where possible by evidence from trials or formal consensus, on the applicability of each therapy to a person with Parkinson's disease at each stage of the disease.

Physiotherapy

The trials of physiotherapy showed some limited evidence of efficacy, particularly with specific gait characteristics such as walking velocity and stride length. Activities of daily living improved in the one trial in which they were measured. Quality of life did not improve in the one trial in which it was measured and economic analysis was not undertaken in any of the trials. The trials used a wide variety of therapy methods, which led to difficulty in determining which type of physiotherapy should be used clinically. The Physiotherapy Evaluation Project (PEP) examined current physiotherapy practice using a Delphi technique, and developed a consensus approach for physiotherapy in Parkinson's disease.[51] Practice guidelines have just been completed by the same group.[9]

Overall, physiotherapy is perceived to be effective in treating balance, gait, posture and mobility, particularly when cueing techniques are used. Early intervention and self-management in the form of a home exercise programme are thought to improve the likelihood of success, followed by frequent (annual) interventions to ensure maintenance of fitness and flexibility. Physiotherapy is perceived to be effective up to the palliative stage of the disease, and even then carers may require physiotherapy to educate them in effective rolling and lifting techniques. A large randomized controlled trial is being designed to examine the effectiveness of physiotherapy using the practice guidelines.

Occupational therapy

The two trials of occupational therapy produced results of little value, due to problems in the design of the trials which could have led to bias, the small numbers of patients examined and the marked heterogeneity of the two methods used. Both trials examined group occupational therapy, which is unlikely to address an individual's specific occupational aims and needs. A Delphi survey to develop a consensus on core occupational therapy practice for Parkinson's disease in the UK has just been completed.[15] Occupational therapists believed that they were generally effective in improving occupational fulfilment at all stages of the disease. As with the physiotherapists, they believed that early and frequent (annual) intervention maximizes potential benefits. This consensus will inform the development of practice guidelines and the design of a large multicentre randomized controlled trial.

Speech and language therapy

The results from the trials of speech and language therapy are encouraging as the improvements measured do appear to be clinically significant. Improved intelligibility must be the primary aim in these trials, however, and this was not measured in the placebo-controlled trials. It should also be noted that much of the data came from two trials that examined the same unique treatment (Lee Silverman Voice Therapy®).[36,38–43] Again, the lack of firm data suggests that a large multicentre randomized controlled trial is required. Although the Royal College of Speech and Language Therapists has published consensus guidelines for the therapy of dysarthria, they are not specific for the treatment of Parkinson's disease and do not contain details of style, duration or intensity of therapy.[10] Speech and language therapists appear to be able to ameliorate some of the communication difficulties experienced by people with Parkinson's disease. Therapy should be provided soon after functional difficulties are noted and followed up on an annual basis. They may also be effective in the treatment of dysphagia but there is very little evidence at any level published in the literature to support this proposition.[52]

Osteopathy

Osteopathy is not generally provided within the NHS so patients have to pay privately for this therapy. The trial of osteopathy was so small that the results can only be used as positive encouragement for the performance of more and larger trials.

The Alexander Technique

The Alexander Technique is another therapy that is purchased privately. However, the results of this trial were very encouraging, particularly in that the improvement in activities of daily living lasted for at least six months. Because the technique educates people with the aim of restoring or maintaining desirable conditions of normality,[53] it is probably applicable across the disease spectrum. A larger trial to examine quality of life and costs will allow a more credible assessment of the benefit of this technique.

Massage

Therapeutic massage is usually provided privately and the results of this trial were not encouraging. No significant benefits were observed but that could have been due to the small size of the trial. A larger trial of therapeutic massage is therefore required for a definitive answer.

Future Trial Design

These reviews emphasize the many methodological shortcomings in the 25 trials of paramedical and complementary therapies in Parkinson's patients, prompting us to make recommendations for conducting future therapy trials in Parkinson's disease and other conditions (Table 3.8). We recognize that the poor quality of

Table 3.8   Recommendations to improve the quality of future paramedical therapy trials

Recommendation	Benefits
Use firm diagnostic criteria, e.g. UK PD Brain Bank Criteria[56]	Excludes patients with Parkinson-plus syndromes
Use clear inclusion and exclusion criteria	Allows enrolment of a uniform cohort of patients
State disease severity of participants, e.g. Hoehn and Yahr score	Allows assessment of which patients benefited most from the therapy and prediction of when best to start therapy
Use large numbers of patients	Reduces selection bias; reduces the chance of false positive or negative results; increases the population of patients to which the results can be applied
Define the therapy method in detail	Allows method to be repeated accurately
Use adequate placebo therapy, i.e. this group should have a similar amount of attention paid to it for the same period of time and in a similar environment as the therapy group	Reduces size of placebo and Hawthorne effects and so strengthens any results
Assess patients for at least six months after therapy	Allows determination of the duration of effect and prediction of how frequently the therapy would have to be repeated to maintain benefits
Note if the patients are 'on' or 'off' when outcomes are measured	Allows clearer assessment of benefits
Use outcomes that have value to patients, e.g. QoL	Allows clearer assessment of benefits
Use outcome scales that are validated, reliable and sensitive in PD	Gives more robust results
Analyse data on an intention-to-treat basis	Reduces bias
Statistically compare changes in outcome measures between the therapy and placebo groups	Correct analysis

UK, United Kingdom; PD, Parkinson's disease; QoL, quality of life.

reporting of some trials may be due to their being published before the adoption of the CONSORT reporting guidelines in 1996.[54] Future reports of trials must conform to these guidelines so that their results can be fairly assessed. Publication bias arises from the tendency for trials with inconclusive or negative results not to be published in peer-reviewed journals. Only one trial out of the 25 reported here found a negative result;[21,22] many trials that found negative or equivocal results may not have been published in peer-reviewed journals. We are aware of at least two unpublished negative trials whose investigators have refused to provide data for analysis in the Cochrane reviews.

Randomized controlled trials of therapies raise some particular difficulties in comparison to trials of drugs. They cannot be double blinded, as both therapist and patient are aware of the therapy allocation. The design of a placebo arm is difficult. Theoretically it should be a neutral intervention that provides as much interpersonal interaction as the therapy itself, in a similar setting and for the same duration. Part of the skill of a therapist, however, lies in maximizing the effect of interpersonal interactions, and so these are as much a part of therapy as, for example, specific exercises. A placebo arm may not be necessary if the design of the trial is pragmatic (see below) and reflects current practice. People with Parkinson's disease often have poor access to paramedical therapies,[14,55–57] so the placebo group could just receive standard care and be untreated by therapists if that is what currently happens. Investigators should be aware of the potential impact of placebo and Hawthorne effects, and effect sizes should be large if they are to be held with confidence.

Large Pragmatic Randomized Controlled Trials

Recent developments in the design of randomized controlled trials have promoted the use of so-called pragmatic trials. These examine the efficacy of current practice healthcare in as realistic a manner as possible. Thus therapies do not have to be tightly prescribed and given only to a very limited patient pool, as has often been the case historically. Instead, patients can be enrolled into the trial on an uncertainty principle: if it is uncertain in the opinion of both the investigator and the patient whether a particular therapy would be of benefit, the patient is randomized to receive it or to receive standard care. The patient then receives an individually tailored course of therapy. In order to make the trial practical, the period of therapy is limited to an average duration.

The primary outcomes are usually quality of life and health economic assessments. This allows the determination of the cost of the intervention as well as the impact on the patient's quality of life. Most assessments are patient completed. This has two benefits, as not only are patients far more accurate in their assessment of their symptoms than the medical professionals but it also reduces the time that a therapist has to spend on the components of the trial rather than standard therapy, keeping the trial closer to real life.

Pragmatic trials could have a large impact in the field of therapy for Parkinson's disease. Such trials would allow the efficacy of each therapy to be assessed at each disease stage. They would also allow an assessment of the real costs of providing the therapy in comparison to medical support alone. These cost analyses should include social as well as medical costs, for social costs may be the area of greatest potential cost savings. The trials could provide a baseline against which all further innovations in the field may be compared. They could also have impact in other areas of therapeutic practice, such as therapies for other neurodegenerative conditions and elderly care. It would also raise the profile of the therapy examined and increase its credibility.

Appendix A

Search method for randomized controlled trials of non-pharmacological therapies for Parkinson's disease.

Relevant trials were identified by electronic searches of up to 21 biomedical databases and clinical trials registers, and an examination of the reference lists of identified studies and other reviews up to the year 2000.

- Biomedical databases: MEDLINE (1966–2000); EMBASE (1974–2000); CINAHL (1982–2000); ISI-SCI ((1981–2000).
- Rehabilitation databases: AMED (1985–2000); MANTIS (1880–2000); REHABDATA (1956–2000); REHADAT and GEROLIT (1979–2000).
- English-language databases of foreign language research and developing world publications: Pascal (1984–2000); LILACS (1982–2000); MedCarib (17th century–2000); JICST-EPlus (1985–2000); AIM (1993–2000), IMEMR (1984–2000).

- Grey literature databases: SIGLE (1980–2000); ISI-ISTP (1982–2000); DISSABS (1999–2000); Conference Papers Index (1982–2000); Aslib Index to Theses (1970–2000).
- Trials registers: Cochrane Controlled Trials Register; CentreWatch Clinical Trials listing service; metaRegister of Controlled Trials; ClinicalTrials.gov; CRISP; PEDro; NIDRR and NRR.

The search terms were divided into three sets of terms linked by OR:

- Set 1: speech; dysarthria; voice; language; dysphagia; swallow; physiotherapy; physical therapy; exercise; occupational therapy; rehabilitation.
- Set 2: osteopathy; Alexander Technique; conductive education; chiropractic; acupuncture; complementary medicine; alternative medicine; massage; holistic health; aromatherapy; biodanza system; tuina; Chinese traditional medicine; yin-yang; integrative medicine.
- Set 3: Parkinson; Parkinson's disease; parkinsonian.

Set 1 was combined with Set 3 with AND, and all the databases listed above were searched.
Set 2 was combined with Set 3 with AND, and only MEDLINE, EMBASE and CINHAL were searched.

Only randomized controlled trials which examined non-pharmacological treatments of Parkinson's disease were included; however, those trials that allowed quasi-random methods of allocation (such as alternate allocation) were allowed.

Appendix B

Criteria for quality assessment

Quality item	Definition
Randomization method	**Adequate** Truly random methods as use of random number tables **Inadequate** Quasi-random methods such as alternate allocation
Concealment of allocation	**Adequate** The allocation of patients into a group was concealed in a manner impervious to any influence by the individual making the allocation, e.g. by having allocation in sealed, opaque sequentially numbered envelopes **Inadequate** The allocation is unconcealed, e.g. list of random numbers was posted on bulletin board
Co-interventions constant (e.g. drug therapy)	**Adequate** Medication was kept constant during the therapy; changes in medication were allowed during the follow-up period **Inadequate** No attempt was made to keep drugs constant
Placebo therapy	**Adequate** Participants were 'treated' with an inactive form of therapy for a similar period of time and in a similar location to the active therapy group **Inadequate** Untreated or treated for a lesser period of time or in a significantly different setting
Withdrawals described and <10% of original population	**Adequate** Reasons for all withdrawals provided; total number of withdrawals less than 10% of the original population **Inadequate** Reasons not given and number withdrawn is greater than 10% of the original population

Quality item	Definition
Blinded assessors	**Adequate** Assessors prevented from knowing allocation of participants **Inadequate** Assessors aware of participant allocation
Missing values present for <10% of original population	**Adequate** Missing values due to incomplete assessment or withdrawals are less than 10% of the original population **Inadequate** Missing values are greater than 10% of the original population
Intention-to-treat data analysis	**Adequate** Data analysed on the basis of randomized allocation irrespective of protocol deviations; missing data substituted by using 'last observation carried forward' **Inadequate** Data analysed on a 'per protocol' basis, according to actual treatment received and ignoring withdrawals
Between group statistical data comparison	**Adequate** Appropriate statistical tests used to compare data between the two treatment groups, either the data at the end time point or the change in the data over the duration of the trial **Inadequate** Inappropriate statistical methods used or the groups not compared statistically one with the other

References

1. Cotzias GC, van Woert HH, Schieffer LM (1967) Aromatic amino acids and modification of parkinsonism. *N Engl J Med* **276**: 374–9.

2. Koller WC, Hubble JP (1990). Levodopa therapy in Parkinson's disease. *Neurology* **40**: 40–7.

3. Cox JCG, Pearce I, Steiger MJ, Pearce JMS (1987) Disordered axial movement in Parkinson's disease. A true apraxia? *Curr Probl Neurol* **6**: 71–5.

4. Lakke JPWF (1985). Axial apraxia in Parkinson's disease. *J Neurol Sci* **69**: 37–46.

5. Steiger MJ, Thompson PD, Marsden CD (1996) Disordered axial movement in Parkinson's disease. *J Neurol Neurosurg Psychiatry* **61**: 645–8.

6. NHS Executive (1997) *Rehabilitation: a guide*. London: HMSO, Department of Health.

7. Wade DT, de Jong BA (2000) Recent advances in rehabilitation. *BMJ* **320** (7246): 1385–8.

8. *Medical Rehabilitation: the Pattern for the Future*. HMSO, Scottish Home and Health Department, Social Health Services Council, London, 1972.

9. *Guidelines for physiotherapy practice in Parkinson's disease*. http://online.unn.ac.uk/faculties/hswe/research/Rehab/Guidelines/intro.htm.

10. Dysarthria. In: van der Gaag A, Reid D, eds. *Clinical Guidelines by Consensus for Speech and Language Therapists*. M and M Press, Glasgow, 1998: 43–8.

11. Burnard P (1989) *Counselling Skills for Health Professionals*. Chapman & Hall, London.

12. www.cot.co.uk

13. Global Parkinson's Disease Survey (2000) *An Insight into Quality of Life with Parkinson's Disease*. The Parkinson's Disease Society of the UK, London.

14. Hurwitz A (1989) The benefit of a home exercise regimen for ambulatory Parkinson's disease patients. *J Neurosci Nurs* **21**(3): 180–4.

15. Deane KHO, Ellis-Hill C, Dekker K *et al.* (2003) A Delphi survey of best practice occupational therapy for Parkinson's disease in the United Kingdom. *Br J Occup Ther* June.

16. Cerri C, Arosio A, Biella AM *et al.* (1994) Physical exercise therapy of Parkinson's. *Mov Disord* **9**(Suppl. 1): 68.

17. Chandler C, Plant R (1999) A targeted physiotherapy service for people with Parkinson's disease from diagnosis to end stage: a pilot study. In: Percival R, Hobson P, eds, *Parkinson's Disease: Studies in psychological and social care*. BPS Books, Leicester: 256–69.

18. Comella CL, Stebbins GT, Brown-Toms N, Goetz CG (1994) Physical therapy and Parkinson's disease: A controlled clinical trial. *Neurology* **44**: 376–8.

19. Forkink A, Toole T, Hirsch MA *et al.* (1996) *The effects of a balance and strengthening program on equilibrium in Parkinsonism.* Florida State University Press, Tallahassee.

20. Toole T, Hirsch MA, Forkink A *et al.* (2000) The effects of a balance and strength training program on equilibrium in Parkinsonism: A preliminary study. *NeuroRehabilitation* **14**(3): 165–74.

21. Gibberd FB, Page NGR, Spencer KM *et al.* (1981) A controlled trial of physiotherapy for Parkinson's disease. In: Rose FC, Capildeo R, eds, *Recent Progress in Parkinson's Disease.* Pitman Medical, Tunbridge Wells: 401–3.

22. Gibberd FB, Page NGR, Spencer KM *et al.* (1981) Controlled trial of physiotherapy and occupational therapy for Parkinson's disease. *BMJ* **282**: 1196.

23. Homann CN, Crevenna R, Kojnig H *et al.* (1998) Can physiotherapy improve axial symptoms in parkinsonian patients? A pilot study with the computerized movement analysis battery Zebris. *Mov Disord* **13**(Suppl. 2): 234.

24. Katsikitis M, Pilowsky I (1996) A controlled study of facial mobility treatment in Parkinson's disease. *J Psychosom Res* **40**(4): 387–96.

25. Schenkman M, Cutson TM, Kuchibhatla M *et al.* (1998) Exercise to improve spinal flexibility and function for people with Parkinson's disease: A randomised controlled trial. *J Am Geriatr Soc* **46**: 1207–16.

26. Thaut MH, McIntosh GC, Rice RR *et al.* (1996) Rhythmic auditory stimulation in gait training for Parkinson's disease patients. *Mov Disord* **11**(2): 193–200.

27. Marchese R, Diverio M, Zucchi F *et al.* (2000) Comparison of two physical therapy approaches in the rehabilitation of parkinsonian patients: a comparison of two physical therapy protocols. *Mov Disord* **15**(5): 879–83.

28. Hirsch MA. *Activity-dependent enhancement of balance following strength and balance training* [doctoral]. Florida State University, Tallahassee.

29. Muller V, Mohr B, Rosin R *et al.* (1997) Short-term effects of behavioral treatment on movement initiation and postural control in Parkinson's disease: A controlled clinical study. *Mov Disord* **12**(3): 306–14.

30. Mohr B, Muller V, Mattes R *et al.* (1996) Behavioral treatment of Parkinson's disease leads to improvement of motor skills and to tremor reduction. *Behav Ther* **27**: 235–55.

31. Palmer SS, Mortimer JA, Webster DD *et al.* (1986) Exercise therapy for Parkinson's disease. *Arch Phys Med Rehab* **67**: 741–5.

32. Shiba Y, Obuchi S, Toshima H, Yamakita H (1999) Comparison between visual and auditory stimulation in gait training of patients with idiopathic Parkinson's disease. *World Congress of Physical Therapy Conference.*

33. Fiorani C, Mari F, Bartolini M *et al.* (1997) Occupational therapy increases ADL score and quality of life in Parkinson's disease. *Mov Disord* **12**(Suppl. 1): 135.

34. Gauthier L, Dalziel S, Gauthier S (1987) The benefits of group occupational therapy for patients with Parkinson's disease. *Am J Occup Ther* **41**(6): 360–5.

35. Johnson JA, Pring TR (1990) Speech therapy and Parkinson's disease: A review and further data. *Br J Disord Commun* **25**: 183–94.

36. Ramig LO, Sapir S, Fox C, Countryman S (2001) Changes in vocal loudness following intensive voice treatment (LSVT) in individuals with Parkinson's disease: A comparison with untreated patients and normal age-matched controls. *Mov Disord* **16**(1): 79–83.

37. Robertson SJ, Thomson F (1984) Speech therapy in Parkinson's disease: a study of the efficacy and long-term effects of intensive treatment. *Br J Disord Commun* **19**: 213–24.

38. Ramig LO, Countryman S, Thompson LL, Horii Y (1995) Comparison of two forms of intensive speech treatment for Parkinson's disease. *J Speech Hear Res* **38**: 1232–51.

39. Ramig LO, Countryman S, O'Brien C *et al.* (1996) Intensive speech treatment for patients with Parkinson's disease: Short- and long-term comparison of two techniques. *Neurology* **47**: 1496–504.

40. Ramig LO, Dromey C (1996) Aerodynamic mechanisms underlying treatment-related changes in vocal intensity in patients with Parkinson's disease. *J Speech Hear Res* **39**: 798–807.

41. Ramig L, Hoyt P, Seeley E, Sapir S (1999) Voice treatment (LSVT) for IPD: Perceptual findings. *Parkinsonism Rel Disord* **5**(Suppl.): S42.

42. Ramig LO, Sapir S, Countryman S *et al.* (2001) Intensive voice treatment (LSVT) for individuals with Parkinson's disease: A 2-year follow-up. *J Neurol Neurosurg Psychiatry* **71**(4): 493–8.

43. Smith ME, Ramig LO, Dromey C *et al.* (1995) Intensive voice treatment in Parkinson's disease: Laryngostroboscopic findings. *J Voice* **9**(4): 453–9.

44. Scott S, Caird FI (1983) Speech therapy for Parkinson's disease. *J Neurol Neurosurg Psychiatry* **46**: 140–4.

45. Scott S, Caird FI, Williams BO (1985) The effect of speech therapy on communication. In: Scott S, Caird FI, Williams BO, eds, *Communication in Parkinson's disease.* Croom Helm, Beckenham: 47–60.

46. Wells MR, Giantinoto S, D'Agate D *et al.* (1999) Standard osteopathic manipulative treatment acutely improves gait performance in patients with Parkinson's disease. *J Am Osteopath Assoc* **99**(2): 92–8.

47. Stallibrass C, Sissons P, Chalmers C, Heritage S (2002) Randomised controlled trial of the Alexander technique for idiopathic Parkinson's disease. *Clin Rehabil* **16**(7): 695–708.

48. Stallibrass C (1997) An evaluation of the Alexander Technique for the management of disability in Parkinson's disease – a preliminary study. *Clin Rehabil* **11**(1): 8–12.

49. Patti F, Reggio A, Nicoletti F *et al.* (1996) Effects of rehabilitation therapy on parkinsonians' disability and functional independence. *J Neurol Rehabil* **10**(4): 223–31.

50. see ref. 15.

51. Plant R, Jones D, Ashburn A *et al.* (2000) *Physiotherapy for people with Parkinson's disease: UK best practice.* Institute of Rehabilitation, Newcastle Upon Tyne.

52. Deane KHO, Whurr R, Clarke CE *et al.* (2001) Non-pharmacological therapies for dysphagia in Parkinson's disease (Cochrane review). *The Cochrane Library.* Update Software, Oxford: CD002816.

53. Alexander FM (2000) *The Universal Constant in Living* 2000 edn. Redwood Books, Wiltshire.

54. Begg C, Cho M, Eastwood S *et al.* (1996) Improving the quality of reporting of randomized controlled trials. The CONSORT statement. *J Am Med Assoc* **276**(8): 637–9.

55. Scott S, Caird FI (1984) The response of the apparent receptive speech disorder of Parkinson's disease to speech therapy. *J Neurol Neurosurg Psychiatry* **47**: 302–4.

56. Mutch WJ, Strudwick A, Roy SK, Downie AW (1986) Parkinson's disease: disability, review and management. *Br Med J (Clin Res Ed)* **293**(6548): 675–7.

57. Yarrow S. Members 1998 survey of the Parkinson's Disease Society of the United Kingdom. In: Percival R, Hobson P, eds (1999) *Parkinson's Disease: studies in psychological and social care.* Leicester: BPS Books: 79–92.

58. Weed D (1990) *What you think is what you get.* Gil Books, Bristol.

4

Developing and Delivering Services

Dorothy Robertson

Introduction

The task of defining neurodegenerative diseases has been likened to defining the continent of Europe: part history, part science and part politics.[1] A similar analogy can be used to describe the current state of service provision for patients with Parkinson's disease (PD) in the UK. Service delivery encompasses both the clinical aspects of what patients and carers need as well as the organizational, political and financial frameworks of how services are delivered. Plain common sense would put clinical aspects at the centre to inform and shape management but in practice historical patterns of service delivery compounded by resource issues have been the main drivers.

Clinical Aspects: Implications for Service Delivery

Incidence and prevalence data

An individual GP will typically have three or four PD patients on their list and come across a new case only every few years. The diagnosis of PD is essentially clinical and can be difficult even in specialist hands and so not surprisingly, experience counts – 91% of patients with idiopathic PD are correctly diagnosed by Queen Square movement disorder specialists[2] as compared with 53% by GPs.[3] Correct diagnosis is a prerequisite for management and it follows that the first step for service delivery must be access to a specialist opinion. The prevalence figures also argue for continued patient access to a specialist service. Health professionals need to see enough patients to understand this complex condition and to develop and maintain their skills.

Advances in drug therapy

Optimal drug therapy is another prerequisite for management and again argues for specialist involvement. We have come a long way from the statement in Brain's 1969 *Diseases of the Nervous System*, 'levodopa in doses of up to 5 grams looks promising.'[4] A description of the range of treatments available for PD is presented in Chapter 1. As can be seen, applying an evolving evidence base for five different classes of PD drugs requires expertise.

Chronic progressive disease

The World Health Organization has prioritized the need for health-care systems to alter their acute focus to meet the challenge of the inexorable rise in chronic disease.[5] The evidence suggests that investing solely in improving medication and technology will have limited impact compared with paying attention to the organization and delivery of care.[5–7] Effective management is characterized by a team approach with professionals working across organizational boundaries, using evidence-based treatment plans with a key worker to co-ordinate.[7] An essential but neglected aspect relates to self-care. Although there is no specific evidence for PD, research across a wide range of chronic conditions highlights the benefits of facilitating self-management, instilling a sense of control and partnership rather than dependency.[8–11] The concept of the 'expert patient' began in the USA, evolving from initial disease-specific experience[10] into generic courses addressing the core problems of living with chronic illness. These issues are listed in Box 4.1. Within the UK, widespread access to user-led self-management courses is a government priority within the NHS plan with implications for PD services.[11]

Response fluctuations

Patients can exhibit pronounced and sudden variations in symptoms and disability throughout the day – a situation unique to PD.

Box 4.1   Core issues generic to chronic illness[11]

1. Knowing how to recognize and act on symptoms
2. Dealing with acute attacks or exacerbations of the disease
3. Making the most effective use of medicines and treatments
4. Comprehending the implications of professional advice
5. Establishing a stable pattern of sleep and rest, and dealing with fatigue
6. Accessing social and other services
7. Managing work and the resources of employment services
8. Accessing chosen leisure activities
9. Developing strategies to deal with the psychological consequences of the illness
10. Learning to cope with other people's responses to their chronic illness

This complicates both the assessment and the delivery of care and has implications for the education of patients, carers, health professionals and care workers.

Complex disease

We have undoubtedly done our patients a disservice by labelling PD a movement disorder. This focus on movement and its drug treatment has arguably been at the expense of addressing the broader complexity of problems experienced daily by patients.

Patients with PD experience impaired cognitive function, disturbed mood, sexual problems, bladder and bowel dysfunction, pain, disturbed sleep and difficulties with activities of daily living. This complex disorder means that a brief medical consultation is limited in its effect.[12,13]

Age and co-morbidity

Since the mean age of onset is in the seventh decade and two-thirds of patients are over 70, services must be accessible to and focused on the special needs of older people. Unfortunately, old age does not come alone and co-morbidity complicates management and medication. Elderly patients also tend to have elderly carers with health and mobility problems of their own.[14] Specialist input needs to take account of the general medical background and work with the network of people who may also be involved within primary care and social services. Although most patients are elderly, the special needs of the one in seven who are diagnosed below the age of 60 and the one in 50 below 40 should not be forgotten.

Clinical Management Scale

The MacMahon and Thomas Four-Stage Clinical Management Scale (Figure 4.1) outlines the different issues that need to be addressed, and the range of services required as the person progresses through the diagnosis, maintenance and complex and palliative stages of the disease.[15]

Diagnosis

The Parkinson Disease Consensus Working Group good practice guidelines[16,17] emphasise the need for specialist confirmation of diagnosis (for the reasons outlined above), yet only 45% of GPs routinely refer.[18] Outpatient waiting lists have been a major factor in non-referral and it behoves secondary care to provide a mechanism for rapid assessment to minimize anxiety and consider treatment. However, waiting lists are not the only factor and ageism is prevalent,[19] with 55% of GPs discriminating by age in their decision to refer.[18] Accuracy of diagnosis is not the only issue – it also matters how the diagnosis is told as this has a measurable impact on quality of life even years later.[13] Whilst providing written information and an early clinical review can help, education needs at diagnosis are generally not well met in primary care or with the traditional outpatient clinic.[14] The process is individual, it takes time and needs to involve carers who may not have attended the clinic. Multidisciplinary input may be required even in this early stage depending on delay in diagnosis and co-morbidity. Access to a PD specialist nurse greatly facilitates the drip-feed of information and counselling which is needed to get this first stage of diagnosis acceptance right.

Maintenance phase

Maintenance is defined as 'keeping a thing in good condition'. As all house and car owners know, maintenance is not just waiting until the problems set in but is an active process that aims to prevent future problems and deal with minor problems before they get out of hand. A similar active, managed maintenance is needed in PD, yet patients are often left to their own devices in the 'honeymoon' period. The pitfalls are obvious. Patients, especially the elderly often expect to get worse and accept increasing slowness or the onset of falls or incontinence as inevitable. Health professionals in primary care are often unaware of the evolving needs of patients and carers and can have similarly low expectations.[14,20] Re-referral is all too often delayed until a crisis is brewing and unhelpful changes in family dynamics have occurred in response to dependency. Maintaining the maintenance phase requires a system for active monitoring with timely intervention.[7] Telephone follow-up can solve the dilemma of monitoring progress whilst avoiding clinic visits if all is well and randomized controlled trials have shown the effectiveness of this approach.[21,22] When combined with the facility for home visits or primary care-based clinics if needed, PD specialist nurse monitoring can keep people away from hospital. Problems can often be sorted in discussion with primary care workers and minor adjustments to PD medication made in consultation with secondary care, releasing precious outpatient slots. Timely intervention is not achieved by the routine six-monthly outpatient review.

A two-way dialogue is needed with patients and carers knowing whom and when to call for advice, combined with a prompt response when directed to the relevant professional. The aims of the maintenance phase are morbidity relief, maintenance of function and self-care and promotion of normal activities. It is also the time to establish relationships with the specialist team and equip patients and carers with the understanding and skills they will need for the future. Generic aspects are important but issues specific to PD also need to be taught. The explosion of access to information via the media and internet has not always been matched by quality, and families should be made aware of reliable

Pathways

A PARADIGM FOR DISEASE MANAGEMENT IN PARKINSON'S DISEASE

Diagnosis

AIMS
Development of disease awareness
Reduction in symptoms and distress
Acceptance of diagnosis

Assessment
(Medical and nursing)
Accurate diagnosis
Evaluate disability
Assess support available
Estimate patient understanding

MANAGEMENT
Develop care plan
Consider multidisciplinary referral
● Specialist nurse
● Physiotherapy
● OT
● Social worker
● Dietician
Assistance & advice with medication
(not always required)
Provide patient/carer education
● Employment
● Driving
● Finances

OUTCOMES
Effective symptom control
Reduced patient distress

Maintenance

AIMS
Morbidity relief
Maintenance of function and self-care
Promotion of normal activities

Re-assessment
Avoid unnecessary medical
dependency
Reduce symptoms
Avoid side-effects
Alert for complications
(e.g. constipation,
postural hypotension)

MANAGEMENT
Review care plan
Provide patient/carer education
Assistance & advice with medication
single or dual drug therapy
Consider multidisciplinary referral
● Speech (and language) therapy
● Physiotherapy
● OT
● Social worker
● Dietician
Assess carer needs
● Benefits
● Support

OUTCOMES
Symptom reduction
Treatment compliance
Maintenance & promotion
of normal activities

Complex

AIMS
Morbidity relief
Maintenance of function and self-care
despite advancing disease
Assistance and adaptation of
environment to promote daily
living activities

Re-assessment
Because of increasing disability
and complexity
Symptom control

MANAGEMENT
Increasingly complex drug
management from disease process
& medication side effects
Advice on practical problems & pre-
vention of complications* (see box)
Referral/liaison may be required
● as in stage I +
● Psychiatrist / CPN
● Neuro-surgery

*Complications
● Motor fluctuations, dyskinesia
● Depression, anxiety
● Self-care, feeding, dysphagia
● Mobility, falls
● Confusion, hallucinations

OUTCOMES
Optimum symptom control
Minimisation of disability
Compliance

Palliative

AIMS
Relief of symptoms and distress in
patients and carer's, morbidity relief
Maintenance of dignity, and remaining
function despite advancing disease
Avoidance of treatment-related
problems

Re-assessment
Symptom control

MANAGEMENT
Advice on administration of
medication
Progressive dopaminergic drug
withdrawal
● Analgesia
● Sedation
Counselling - psychology/psychiatry
Prevention and treatment of
complications
● Urinary incontinence
● Pressure sores
● Motor fluctuations

OUTCOMES
Absence of distress
Maintenance of dignity
Symptoms controlled

Health Gain   Health Maintenance   Comfort

Figure 4.1   MacMahon and Thomas Four-Stage Clinical Management Scale.

PARKINSON'S DISEASE

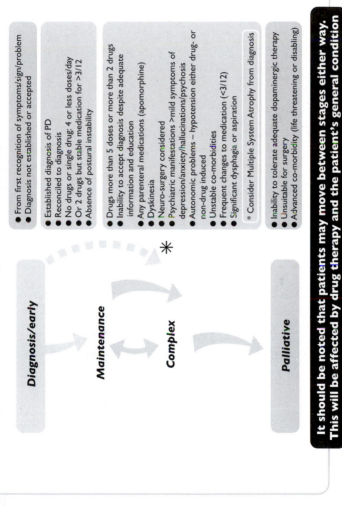

Diagnosis/early
- From first recognition of symptoms/sign/problem
- Diagnosis not established or accepted

Maintenance
- Established diagnosis of PD
- Reconciled to diagnosis
- No drugs or single drug: 4 or less doses/day
- Or 2 drugs but stable medication for >3/12
- Absence of postural instability

Complex
- Drugs more than 5 doses or more than 2 drugs
- Inability to accept diagnosis despite adequate information and education
- Any parenteral medications (apomorphine)
- Dyskinesia
- Neuro-surgery considered
- Psychiatric manifestations >mild symptoms of depression/anxiety/hallucinations/psychosis
- Autonomic problems – hypotension either drug- or non-drug induced
- Unstable co-morbidities
- Frequent changes to medication (<3/12)
- Significant dysphagia or aspiration

* Consider Multiple System Atrophy from diagnosis

Palliative
- Inability to tolerate adequate dopaminergic therapy
- Unsuitable for surgery
- Advanced co-morbidity (life threatening or disabling)

It should be noted that patients may move between stages either way. This will be affected by drug therapy and the patient's general condition

Figure 4.1 (cont.)

Source: MacMahon DG, Thomas S. Practical approach to quality of life in Parkinson's Disease. *Journal of Neurology* (1998) 245 [Suppl I]: S19–S22.

sources such as the Parkinson's Disease Society. PD group exercise and education sessions improve patient and carer understanding of the disease and its treatment and are a useful means of conveying and re-enforcing the principles that underpin PD rehabilitation strategies.[23] This approach is used in many multidisciplinary specialist services and is highly valued by participants although there is a need for formal evaluation and some individual input may also be required. The PD service in Guildford has produced an information pack for patients and professionals outlining the structure and content of their programme – a useful resource for clinics planning to start group courses.[23]

Complex phase

Management in the established complex phase can be a difficult balancing act with competing and often opposing priorities: increased medication for mobility at the expense of hallucinations, confusion or falls; improved control versus greater drug complexity; and conflict between the needs and views of patients and carers. Brokering compromise takes time and is helped if a basis of trust and communication has been established earlier in the illness. Health professionals, carers and care workers require education to enable them to recognize, understand and manage the differing care needs when 'on' and 'off'. Getting the drugs right is essential with monitoring for side effects and access for urgent review when things go wrong.

The PD specialist nurse role is ideally suited to facilitate compliance with often complicated drug regimes and provide education and urgent advice. In addition, the breadth of symptomatology and the frequency of problems with practical tasks in daily life dictate a team approach so that problems that doctors do not have the training or time to deal with are addressed, with a key worker (usually the PD specialist nurse) to direct the traffic and ensure co-ordinated care and communication. The need for specialist team management is strongly supported by consensus guidelines[16,17] but for most patients it is simply rhetoric. Surveys show that up to 70% of patients with PD have no regular contact with secondary care and rely entirely on their general practitioners.[24–26]

Access to therapists is also generally poor in the UK.[14,24,27,28] In 1998, only 20% of PD Society members had ever seen a speech therapist, 27% a physiotherapist and 17% an occupational therapist. These figures overestimate the number of patients receiving therapy as part of chronic disease management as it includes ever seeing a therapist for anything. The difference between multidisciplinary input and co-ordinated interdisciplinary team care should also be emphasized (Table 4.1).[29,30] A recent Delphi survey of current occupational therapy practice in the UK highlights the paradox that patients in the more advanced stages of the disease are more likely to be seen by a social services OT working usually in isolation.[33]

Table 4.1 Problems at night

Multidisciplinary input	• medical review of medication – **next outpatient appointment in 3 months** • District Nurse assessment of continence • referred to social services for OT input – **classed as non-urgent** • seen by domiciliary physiotherapist – **not yet seen by OT** • assess impact on carer and advise re allowances, care and respite – **not done, whose job?**
Interdisciplinary management	Team assessment and discussion of problems with agreed action plan for: • medical review of medication • mental health input as agitated with depression and recent hallucinations • joint medical and nursing assessment of continence problems – agree management plan with patient, carer and District Nurse • joint physiotherapy and occupational therapy assessment of bed mobility, review technique and re-enforce movement strategies; discuss with carer • OT advice regarding equipment • nursing input to avoid pressure sores • social work assessment of impact on carer; advice regarding attendance allowance, care agencies and respite care • key worker to co-ordinate Reassessment and team discussion Face-to-face discussion and use of shared notes

Palliative care

The relief of symptoms and distress for patients and carers and the retention of dignity are the main aims of this phase with a shift in emphasis from drugs to nursing aspects and the provision of equipment, appropriate care and emotional support. Primary care plays an increasing role, especially the District Nurse who should be supported by specialist input from the PD service, mental health or the local hospice as needed. This means access to telephone advice and the facility for domiciliary visits if needed. The palliative management of PD has received little attention, both clinically and in terms of research. Patients are often discharged when clinic attendance is no longer practical with primary care and the family being left to get on with it.

Current provision of services: the needs/care mismatch

Why is there such a mismatch between what is needed and what happens in practice? Some of the issues are listed in the box below. Our current healthcare system evolved in response to acute, mainly infectious illness which has left its mark in terms of organization and attitude. In PD there has been a single-minded and somewhat naïve focus on drugs as a kind of Holy Grail. Undergraduate and postgraduate education must reflect the change in the burden of disease from short-lived acute to chronic, with a

---

Box 4.2   Service/needs mismatch: contributing factors

- Acute focused health system
- Underprovision of movement disorder specialists (including specialist therapists and nurses)
- Limitations of traditional medical outpatient model of care
- Doctors as gatekeepers to multidisciplinary input
- Lack of key worker to co-ordinated chronic disease management within specialist team
- Research focus on impairment rather than quality of life
- Therapeutic focus on movement rather than quality of life
- Emphasis on waiting list initiatives rather than changing the system

corresponding change in research emphasis to focus on factors that impact on quality of life.[5,12,13,31]

Why is patient access to therapists so valued by patients but yet so limited? One factor is underprovision, compounded by the lack of research funding and focus to provide the evidence base for purchasers. The current system for patient referral also acts as a barrier rather than facilitating input. In most areas it is the doctor who acts as gatekeeper to other health professionals working at the disability/handicap end of the spectrum, yet doctors are poor at recognizing patients' functional problems and lack the necessary time and skills.[20] Doctors are also poor at recognizing the value of specialist training within other disciplines, referring to a physiotherapist or occupational therapist without knowledge of or support for their expertise in movement disorders. The recent Delphi surveys of physiotherapists[32] and occupational therapists[33] show that most therapists gain their knowledge by hands-on experience with very little access to training.

Specialist medical input is also limited by underprovision. The Association of British Neurologists report *Acute Neurological Emergencies in Adults, 2002* highlights the lack of consultant neurologists.[34] At persent there are 358 neurologists in the UK (approximately one per 177 000 population), which compares very unfavourably with other European countries (e.g. France one per 38 462; Italy one per 8117; Netherlands one per 25 773). Approximately 75% of neurologists are based in large neurology centres with only 25% being based in local District General Hospitals,[35] an arrangement that re-enforces the isolated medical outpatient model as it is difficult to establish community links from a regional centre.

The underprovision of neurologists in the UK has led, by default, to an increasing expertise in movement disorders within geriatric medicine supported by multidisciplinary educational initiatives from the PD section of the British Geriatric Society. One positive aspect of this broadening of the specialist medical input into both PD patient care and research has been the grounding of Geriatric practice within the context of interdisciplinary teams with the focus on rehabilitation and established networks of communication with primary care. Geriatrician care is also better placed to deal with the frail elderly patient with co-morbidity. The two specialities have a lot to learn from each other and patients gain from close working between them. Within geriatric medicine, a formal

movement disorders training programme (including two-day resi-
dential modules combined with mentorship) was established in the
Autumn of 2002 for consultants running PD clinics and final year
specialist registrars planning to specialize. A similar or joint initia-
tive is needed for neurology to provide training in interdisciplinary
aspects of care.

In 1999, the median wait for a routine neurology outpatient's
appointment varied from 12 weeks in North-East Thames (figures
exclude the National Hospital for Neurology and Neurosurgery) to
51 weeks in Northern Ireland with a maximum of 110.[36] The
emphasis has been on working harder with various waiting list initiatives to try to sort out the problem. Consultant expansion is
clearly needed but will take time. In the meantime, the conclusion
of the US Institute of Medicine regarding the 'quality chasm' in
healthcare is relevant: 'trying harder will not work – changing the
system will.'[37]

Parkinson's disease nurse specialist (PDNS) role

Most effective chronic disease interventions involve specialist
nurses to co-ordinate, ensure adherence to clinical protocols, and
provide education – and this key nursing role is recognized in the
NHS plan.[38,39] The PD Society nurse specialist project was
launched in 1994 based on the experience of the initial appointment in Cornwall in 1989.[40,41] Around 120 nurses – facilitated by
a variety of funding sources including commercial, charitable and
the NHS – are currently in the post. The PD Society aims to recruit
a minimum of 240 to reduce the geographical inequity of provision
and is pump-priming new appointments provided there is a firm
commitment to continued funding. PDNS are employed at a
minimum of G grade rising to H with experience but the role fits
within the Senior Registered Practitioner level within the new
career framework for nurses with the option of Consultant
Practitioner grade.

Differing practice models have evolved depending on local
circumstances as follows.

Hospital-based PDNS

The short-term benefits of this model were evaluated in 108
patients over a year in a randomized comparison of PDNS care
compared with a consultant neurologist. Patients and carers valued

the role suggesting an impact on quality of life but cost-effectiveness was questioned because of similar physical outcomes and increased costs associated with PDNS providing additional care.[42]

Community model

A primary care-based model of care was evaluated in a two-year randomized controlled study of PDNS care compared with ordinary care arranged through the GP.[43] The trial has been criticized as potentially underestimating benefit for several reasons.[44,45] Nurses were evaluated over the first two years of their appointment when still on their learning curve of experience. They also varied in their access to any specialist support as this depended on the local secondary care situation and the degree to which they were welcomed as 'part of the team'. The study also included a large proportion of early stage patients (50% less than five years' duration; 84% on monotherapy; and 34% under the age of 70) in whom a two-year follow-up may be too short to show benefit. Significant improvement in physical outcomes were not demonstrated but nurse input preserved patient well-being at no extra cost.[43]

Integrated health and social care model

In the Parkinson's Disease Forum project[46] (awarded the Beacon Award for Good Practice), a District Nurse with special training in PD became a link person between primary and secondary care, supported by PD consultant clinics held within a health centre. Sixty patients were identified at the start of the project, and medication benefits were maximized or side-effects minimized in 30%. The role of the PDNS was of significant benefit to 25% of patients and the diagnosis altered in 8%. Over the first 18 months of the project four patients avoided care home placement with a saving to social services of £51 000, and a £22 000 saving to a self-funded patient.

Other service models have developed in response to local ideas and geography. The Worcestershire area has opted to develop a network of Community and District Nurses with ENB A43 course training in PD, and the James Parkinson Centre in Cornwall is seeking to establish a similar network but supported by a fully trained PDNS with links to secondary care.

Wherever the PDNS is based, the crucial factor seems to be the facility to move physically between primary and secondary care

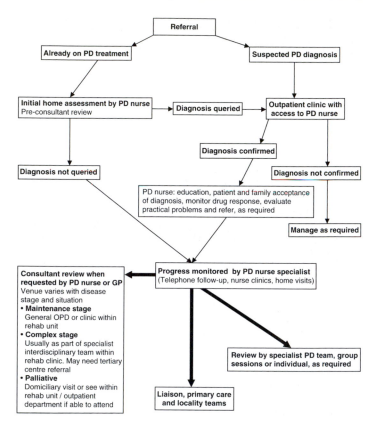

Figure 4.2   Integrated model of PD care.

depending on need with face-to-face contact with specialists and primary care staff.

Political framework

The change in government focus from acute to chronic, reflected in recent policy documents (see Box 4.3), provides a positive framework for commissioning PD services in the future. In common with many neurological disabilities, service needs cut across the artificial departmental boundaries of local authorities, social services and health. The emphasis on partnership and integration is welcome

- *The NHS Plan.* http://www.doh.gov.uk/nhsplan/index.htm
- *The New NHS: modern, dependable.* DOH 1997
- EL(97)62 27 CI(97)24: *Better Service For Vulnerable People*
- *Our Healthier Nation: Saving Lives.* DOH 1999
- *Caring About Carers: a national strategy for carers.* HMSO 1999. http:// www.carers.gov.uk/
- HSC1999/242: LAC (99)38 *Modernising Health and Social Services – National Priorities Guidance 2000/01–2002/03*
- HSC 2001/01: LAC (2001)1 *Intermediate Care*
- HSC 2001/03: LAC (2001)4 *Implementing the NHS Plan: Developing services following the National Beds Inquiry*
- HSC 2001/06: LAC(2001)6 *Better Care Higher Standards: Guidance for 2001/02*
- HSC(2001)008: LAC(2001)013 *Community Equipment Services: Guide to integrating community equipment services*
- The New NHS: Guidance on out – of – area treatment consultation. http://www.doh.gov.uk/nhsexec/ecr.htm
- DOH Guidance on Joint Investment Plans. www.doh.gov.uk/jointunit/jipguidance.htm
- Implementation programme for the NHS Plan. www.doh.gov.uk/nhsplanimpprogramme
- Planning for health and social care: guidance for health and local authorities on service and financial frameworks. www.doh.gov.uk/ nhsplanimpprogramme/planning.htm
- NSF for Older People. www.doh.gov.uk/nsf/pdfs/nsfolderpeople.pdf
- NSF for Longterm Conditions. www.doh.gov.uk/nsf/longterm.htm
- Pharmacy in the future – implementing the NHS plan: a programme for pharmacy in the National Health Service. www.doh.gov.uk/pharmacyfuture/index.htm#top

and has been accompanied by legislative changes to facilitate joint working.[47] The year 1999 saw the transition from Fundholding General Practices into Primary Care Groups. These have now largely evolved into Primary Care Trusts responsible for commissioning services in discussion with Strategic Health Authorities and acute NHS Trusts. The White Paper *The New NHS: modern, dependable*[47] describes the new commissioning arrangements based on Longterm Service Agreements within the context of agreed Health Improvement Plans and Joint Investment Plans, which should link, where relevant, to the new National Service Frameworks (NSFs).[48–51] Care Trusts, the next stage in integration, are beginning to come on-line with the first four in place in April 2002 with a further ten anticipated over the next year.

The NSF for Older People[50] and the new National Strategy for Carers[52] contain much of relevance to people with PD including 'a single assessment process, integrated commissioning arrangements and integrated provision of care.'[50] The key themes that will underpin the NSF for Longterm Conditions (due 2004) are emerging from the consultation process;[51] other documents of relevance to commissioning for PD services are listed in the box below. These can mostly be accessed through the Department of Health web site at http://www.doh.gov.uk/publications/wgpaper.html. The political rhetoric is encouraging but achieving the financial framework for change requires local champions to make the case and get PD services on the agenda.

Box 4.4   Consultation on NSF for Longterm Conditions – key themes[51]

Service users
- Integrated approach within health (primary and secondary care) and between health and social services
- Users at centre of decisions about their care
- Adopt principles of the expert patient, recognizing when not possible or desirable
- Seamless service with continuity of care
- Interdisciplinary approach with single assessment procedure and pathways for different phases of the condition – key worker to co-ordinate
- Equitable access to flexible range of services
- Symptom management – help with range of common symptoms
- Improved community equipment services with equity of access and consumer involvement
- Equal access to welfare, benefits, financial advice, suitable housing, employment, vocational training, transport and leisure services
- Mechanisms to allow regular invitations for review – 'the case that doesn't close'; reviews that users/patients can initiate and mechanism for self-referral to specialist services, e.g. physiotherapy

Box 4.4   Continued

Carers
- User needs assessment without assuming informal carer help
- Pro-active support to prevent carers 'going under'
- Rapid response to change in carer circumstances
- Information about services
- Increased use planned respite
- Recognition of needs of ageing carers

Professional staff
- Integrated health and social care teams with single assessment procedures and review mechanisms
- Continuity of care
- Whole systems approach
- Key workers needed
- Senior managers responsible for implementing NSF
- Review role of GP as gate keeper – seen as a barrier
- Clinical networks of GPs with specialist expertise
- Training

Other government departments
- Links to other relevant policy areas, e.g. transport, benefits and housing

Underpinning issues
- Research and development
- Information – patients, policy makers and managers
- Human resources
- Finance
- Securing and monitoring service delivery
- Project management and process issues

Making the case for investment in Parkinson's disease

Studies suggest an average PCT population of 100 000 will need to commission and provide services for 168 patients with up to 26 new cases being diagnosed each year[53,54] with estimated direct costs of £560 000 to £1.6 million.[55] The document *Moving and*

Shaping – the future. Commissioning Services for People with Parkinson's Disease[55] provides a very useful starting point for discussion. Interested allies should be identified including the voluntary sector, social services, people with PD and carers. Local services are often patchy in quantity and quality. Setting up a task force to perform an initial local service mapping exercise in consultation with the primary care trust Clinical Governance Lead and relevant commissioning managers provides the information and makes the strategic links to move PD services up the priority list.

Access to tertiary care is essential for the diagnostic conundrums and patients with particularly complex problems but, in keeping with other chronic conditions, the routine management of PD requires a firm grounding in primary care, which is best placed to be aware of intercurrent problems and the interplay between medical and social aspects. The PD nurse specialist role is key to providing the integration between local specialist interdisciplinary teams, social services, patients, carers and the voluntary sector envisaged by the relevant National Service Frameworks.

References

1. Williams A (2002) Defining neurodegenerative disease. *BMJ* **324**: 1465–6.
2. Hughes AJ, Daniel SE, Ben-Schlomo Y, Lees AJ (2002) The accuracy of diagnosis of parkinsonian syndromes in a specialist movement disorder service. *Brain* **125** (Pt 4): 861–70.
3. Meara J, Bhowmick BK, Hobson P (1999) Accuracy of diagnosis in patients with presumed Parkinson's disease. *Age Ageing* **28**: 99–102.
4. Brian Lord, Walton J, eds (1969) *Brain's Diseases of the Nervous System*, 7th edn. Oxford University Press, London.
5. Epping-Jordan J, Bengoa R, Kawar R, Sabate E (2001) The challenge of chronic conditions: WHO responds. *BMJ* **323**: 947–8.
6. Stroke Unit Trialists' Collaboration (1997) Collaborative systematic review of the randomised trials of organised inpatient (stroke unit) care after stroke. *BMJ* **314**: 1151–9.
7. Wagner EH (1998) Chronic disease management: what will it take to improve care for chronic illness? *Eff Clin Pract* **1**: 2–4.
8. Lorig KR, Sobel DS, Stewart AL *et al.* (1999) Evidence suggesting that a chronic disease self-management program can improve health status whilst reducing hospitalisation: a randomised trial. *Med Care* **37**(1): 5–14.
9. Lorig KR, Sobel DS, Ritter PL *et al.* (2001) Effect of a self management program on patients with chronic disease. *Eff Clin Pract* **4**(6): 256–62.

10. Shoor S, Lorig KR. Self care and the doctor–patient relationship. *Med Care* **40**(Suppl 4): 1140–4.

11. Department of Health (2001) The expert patient: a new approach to chronic disease management for the 21st century. Department of Health, London. www.ohn.gov.uk/ohn/people/expert.

12. Findley LJ, Baker MG (2002) Treating neurodegenerative diseases. What patients want is not what doctors focus on. *BMJ* **324**: 1466–7.

13. Findley LJ, for the Global Parkinson's Disease Steering Committee (2002) Factors impacting on quality of life in Parkinson's disease: results from an international survey. *Mov Disord* **17**:60–67.

14. Yarrow S (1999) Members' 1998 survey of the Parkinson's Disease Society of the United Kingdom. In: Percival R, Hobson P, eds, *Parkinson's Disease: Studies in Psychological Care*. BPS Books, Leicester: 79–92.

15. MacMahon D, Thomas S (1998) Practical approach to quality of life in Parkinson's disease. *J Neurol* **245** (Suppl. 1): S19–S22.

16. Bhatia K, Brooks DJ, Burn DJ *et al.* (1998) Guidelines for the management of Parkinson's disease. The Parkinson's Disease Consensus Working Group. *Hosp Med* **59**(6): 469–80.

17. Bhatia K, Brooks DJ, Burn DJ *et al.* (2001) Parkinson's Disease Consensus Working Group. Updated guidelines for the management of Parkinson's disease. *Hosp Med* **62**(8): 456–70.

18. MacMahon DG, Baker M, Primary Care Task Force (1999) *Parkinson's Aware in Primary Care*, 2nd edn. Parkinson's Disease Society, London.

19. Lothian K, Philp I (2001) Maintaining the dignity and autonomy of older people in the healthcare setting. *BMJ* **322** (7287): 668–70.

20. Koplas PA, Gans HB, Wisely MP, *et al.* (1999) Quality of life and Parkinson's disease. *J Gerontol A Biol Sci Med Sci* **54**(4): M197–M202.

21. Von Korff M, Gruman J, Schaefer J *et al.* (1997) Collaborative management of chronic illness. *Ann Int Med* **127**(12): 1097–102.

22. Wasson J, Gaudette C, Whaley F *et al.* (1992) Telephone care as a substitute for routine clinic follow-up. *JAMA* **267**: 1828–29.

23. Trend P, Kaye J (2001) Multidisciplinary Care in Parkinson's Disease and Parkinsonism – From Science to Practice. The British Geriatric Society PD Section. 6th National Conference. Royal College of Physicians, London.

24. Mutch WJ, Strudwick A, Roy SK, Downie AW (1986) Parkinson's disease: disability, review, and management. *BMJ* **293**: 675–7.

25. College of Health (1994) *The needs of people with Parkinson's disease*. College of Health, London.

26. Ridsdale L (1995) Community care for patients with idiopathic Parkinson's disease. *Br J Gen Pract* **394**: 226–7.

27. Oxtoby M (1982) *Parkinson's disease patients and their social needs*. Parkinson's Disease Society, London.

28. Clarke CE, Zobkiw RM, Gullaksen E (1995) Quality of life and care in Parkinson's disease. *Br J Clin Pract* **49**: 288–93.

29. Melvin JL (1980) Interdisciplinary and multidisciplinary activities and ACRM. *Arch Phys Med Rehabil* **61**: 379–80.

30. Davis A, Davis S, Moss N (1992) First steps towards an interdisciplinary approach to rehabilitation. *Clin Rehabil* **6**: 237–44.

31. Janca A (1999) A report on the WHO Working Group on Parkinson's Disease. *Neuroepidemiology* **18**: 236–40.

32. Guidelines for physiotherapy practice in Parkinson's disease. http://online.unn.ac.uk/faculties/hswe/research/Rehab/Guidelines/intro.htm.

33. Deane KHO, Ellis-Hill C, Dekker K *et al.* (2003) A Delphi survey of best practice occupational therapy for Parkinson's disease in the United Kingdom. *Br J Occup Ther* June.

34. Association of British Neurologists (2002) *Acute Neurological Emergencies in Adults, 2002.* Ormond House, 27 Boswell St, London WC1N 3JZ, UK; http://www.theabn.org/.

35. Association of British Neurologists (1997) *Neurology in the United Kingdom towards 2000 and beyond.* 27 Boswell St, London WC1N 3JZ, UK; http://www.theabn.org/.

36. Association of British Neurologists web site http://www.theabn.org/.

37. Institute of Medicine (2001) *Crossing the quality chasm: a new health system for the 21st century.* National Academy Press, Washington DC.

38. Wagner EH (2000) The role of patient care teams in chronic disease management. *BMJ* **320**: 569–72.

39. HM Government (2000) *The NHS Plan.* HMSO, London.

40. Parkinson's Disease Nurse Specialist Association web site http://www.pdnsa.org.uk.

41. Parkinson's Disease Society (1999) *Parkinson's Disease and the Nurse.* Parkinson's Disease Society, London.

42. Reynolds H, Wilson-Barnett J, Richardson G (2000) Evaluation of the role of the Parkinson's disease nurse specialists. *Int J Nurs Stud* **37**: P337–P339.

43. Jarman B, Hurwitz B, Cook A, *et al.* (2002) Effects of community-based nurses specialising in Parkinson's disease on health outcome and costs: a randomised controlled trial. *BMJ* **324**: 1072–5.

44. Clarke CE, MacMahon DG, Findley LJ, (2002) Parkinson's Disease Nurse Specialists (letter). *BMJ* **324**.

45. Huyse F, de Jonge P, Slaets JPJ (2002) Appropriate patient selection and training are needed for Parkinson nurse specialist (letter). *BMJ* **324**.

46. Dunstan C, Castledon B (1999); BAMM Hospital Doctor medical management team of the year awards.

47. *The new NHS: modern, dependable* (1997) Department of Health; http://www.doh.gov.uk/publications/wgpaper.html.

48. HSC1999/242, LAC (99)38 Modernising Health and Social Services – National Priorities Guidance 2000/01–2002/03.
49. Department of Health. Guidance on Joint Investment Plans; http://www.doh.gov.uk/jointunit/jipguidance.htm.
50. NSF for older people; http://www.doh.gov.uk/nsf/pdfs/nsfolder-people.pdf.
51. NSF for long-term conditions; http://www.doh.gov.uk/nsf/longterm.htm.
52. HMSO (1999) *Caring about carers: a national strategy for carers.* http://www.carers.gov.uk/.
53. Cockerell OC, Goodridge DM, Brodie D *et al.* (1996) Neurological disease in the defined population: the results of a pilot study in two general practices. *Neuroepidemiology* **15**: 73–82.
54. Schrag A, Ben-Schlomo Y, Quinn NP (2000) Cross-sectional prevalence survey of Parkinson's disease and parkinsonism in London. *BMJ* **321**: 21–2.
55. Thomas S, MacMahon, Henry S (1999) *Moving and Shaping – the future. Commissioning services for people with Parkinson's disease.* Parkinson's Disease Society UK, Primary Care Task Force, London.

5

Evaluating the Outcome of Rehabilitation Interventions

Ray Fitzpatrick

Introduction

Parkinson's disease (PD) is a chronic degenerative neurological disease with a prevalence of just over 1 per 1000 and increasing incidence at older ages. Clinical assessment has conventionally emphasized the distinguishing functional problems such as tremor, rigidity, bradykinesia and postural instability. However, the disease has a wider potential impact on individuals so that evaluation of outcomes of interventions has increasingly gone beyond clinical assessments to take account of the broader impact of PD on health-related quality of life. Wherever possible this broader approach relies on patients' own assessments through self-completed questionnaires and related methods.

Clinical Scales

The simplest clinical scale to assess PD, devised by Hoehn and Yahr, distinguishes between five stages of severity of the disease from (stage 1) unilateral involvement with minimal or no functional impairment to (stage 5) confined to wheelchair or bed.[1] It is still the most widely used rating scale to describe samples for the purposes of comparison but it is too crude and insensitive to be useful as a measure of outcomes of interventions.

As the need for assessment of interventions has grown, over 20 other clinical rating scales have been developed to assess the core impact of PD.[2] They typically focus upon ratings by the clinician of the core signs of tremor, rigidity, gait abnormalities and, to a lesser extent, functional abilities such as walking and feeding. Few of the scales require that the clinician assess any broader emotional or social impact of PD. Many of the scales have received little or no examination in terms of basic measurement properties such as reliability and validity.

The diverse content and methods of scoring of the array of available scales has made comparison of studies and meta-analysis of interventions problematic. To address the plurality of clinical rating scales, a concerted effort was made to produce a 'gold-standard' measure resulting, in 1987, with the Unified Parkinson's Disease Rating Scale (UPDRS). This is composed of subscales to assess mental, motor and activities of daily living scores, a section on the complications of dopaminergic therapy, and a modified Hoehn and Yahr scale.[3] Research appears occasionally proposing modifications to the UPDRS which are intended to improve its measurement properties.[4] Sensitivity to change over time is still formally underexamined although extensive evidence from its use in trials exists.

In a systematic review of randomized drug trials for PD between 1966 and 1998 it was found that by far the most commonly used disease-specific scale (33% of trials) was the UPDRS.[5]

By comparison, the more recently developed generic health status measures (discussed below) were used in 3% of trials. Overall, the UPDRS has been the most thoroughly developed clinical scale in outcome measurement in PD.

Two related developments have broadened the approach taken to assessing outcomes of interventions for PD. Firstly it has become increasingly clear that this disease has a wide range of potential effects on individuals not directly addressed by clinical scales such as the UPDRS. Such problems might include social isolation and lack of support from spouse or family, embarrassment and concerns about others' reaction to PD, fears of falling, feelings of anger or worry about the future. In a study of such patients attending a

PD clinic, one of the largest differences in reported problems (compared with matched control groups) was in relation to social isolation.[6] In a second, similarly designed study one of the biggest differences in patients with PD compared with matched controls was in the greater frequency with which patients with PD reported problems controlling their voice and being able to speak clearly.[7]

Secondly it has become apparent that, even where scales such as the UPDRS do include items addressing particular consequences of PD, they may more accurately and efficiently be reported by patients rather than be mediated by clinical judgements of the nature and severity of problems. Agreement between clinician and patient is greater for more observable aspects of health status such as performance of activities of daily living but reduces as more personal consequences of health such as emotional well-being become salient.[8,9] Discrepancies in judgements between patients and health professionals are commonly observed for other neurological disorders and for health problems more generally.[10,11]

A growing emphasis in all fields of medicine has been wherever possible to make the patient the judge of personal aspects of health status and health-related quality of life.

Three different kinds of measures have been developed to enable the patient to judge health-related quality of life:

- generic health status measures
- disease-specific measures
- utility or preference measures.

All three types of measure have been applied as outcome measures in neurology.

Generic health status measures

As their name implies, these instruments have been developed to be relevant to the widest possible range of health problems, so that results of studies can be applied across diverse types of health problems, e.g. comparing levels of need or the effectiveness of interventions across diseases and types of intervention. Because questions are general in intent, they can also be completed by general community samples, providing the opportunity to compare health profiles of specific patient groups – such as patients with PD – with community 'norms' or average population values.

The Nottingham Health Profile

An early example of this is the Nottingham Health Profile (NHP).[12] The core of the NHP comprises 38 statements to which respondents select 'Yes' or 'No'. Individual items are weighted to reflect severity of item and contribute to one of six dimensions: emotional reactions; energy; pain; physical mobility; sleep; and social isolation. The NHP has been extensively tested for reliability and validity prior to its use in PD research. In a community survey of PD in Norway, respondents with PD had poorer scores than age-matched controls for all dimensions of the NHP, but particularly poor scores for physical mobility, energy and sleep.[13] In multivariate analysis, it was striking that respondents' overall health-related quality of life scores were more strongly related to depressive symptoms and disability scores than to the clinical UPDRS motor subscale. Followed up four years later, the NHP scores had further deteriorated with regard to physical mobility, emotional reactions, pain and social isolation.[14] The presence of depressive symptoms and disability continued to be better predictors of health-related quality of life as reflected in the total NHP score. The authors conclude with concern that, despite readily available modern healthcare, health-related quality of life substantially declines in a community-representative sample of individuals with PD over a four-year period.

The NHP has been used to evaluate interventions for PD. For example, Sitzia *et al.,* in an uncontrolled longitudinal study, provided 5 to 10-day multidisciplinary inpatient rehabilitation for patients with both PD and multiple sclerosis, and observed significantly improved NHP total scores one month after discharge.[15]

The Medical Outcomes Study 36-item Short Form

Another generic health status instrument, the Medical Outcomes Study 36-item Short Form (SF-36) was developed after the NHP.[16] It has subsequently become the most widely used of all generic health status measures.[17]

> The SF-36 comprises 36 questions, which contribute to eight
> dimensions: physical function; role physical; bodily pain;
> general health perceptions; vitality; social function; mental
> health; and role emotional.

Two summary scores can also be derived: physical and mental components. The SF-36 was used to assess respondents with PD in a community survey in Finland.[18] Results indicated that PD had its most adverse effects on the more physical aspects of health-related quality of life compared to social and emotional aspects of well-being, which were less influenced by PD. In multivariate analyses, for most dimensions of SF-36, depressive symptoms were a greater predictor of poor scores than was Hoehn and Yahr, the exception being physical functioning where the reverse held.

Chrischilles *et al.* used SF-36 with patients with PD attending a clinic in Iowa, USA, and found that, although clinical measures from the UPDRS were helpful in explaining much of the variance in SF-36 physical function, they did not explain much of the variation for other dimensions of SF-36.[19] As with studies of the NHP, mental health seemed a more important predictor of other aspects of health-related quality of life scores in SF-36. Gray *et al.* used SF-36 to assess the impact of a range of neurosurgical procedures on quality of life for patients with PD before and three months after surgery.[20] They found greater beneficial effects as reflected in SF-36 for unilateral and bilateral pallidotomy than were obtained from unilateral thalamotomy but recognized that patient selection and non-randomized study design made such differences difficult to interpret.

Disease-specific measures

It is increasingly recognized that generic health status measures may not be sensitive to the specific health problems and outcomes associated with a specific disease, hence the emergence of so-called disease-specific measures. Four such measures have been developed for use in PD as follows.

The Parkinson's Impact Scale

Calne *et al.* developed the Parkinson's Impact Scale (PIMS) by inviting health professionals to design a scale, and then testing it on patients.[21] The resulting scale has ten items covering self, feelings, family, community, work, travel, leisure, financial security, safety and sexuality, with respondents rating on a four-point scale the severity of impact of PD. Factor analysis identified four underlying dimensions: physical; social; psychological; and financial. It would appear that this instrument depends on some degree of health professional advice and support to be completed satisfactorily. The authors examined construct validity by establishing poorer scores for the instrument during 'off' states.

The Parkinson's Disease Quality of Life Questionnaire

De Boer *et al.* in the Netherlands developed the Parkinson's Disease Quality of Life Questionnaire (PDQL) selecting items as a result of open-ended interviews with patients and neurologists.[22] Seventy-three items were initially identified in this way and the final 37-item version selected from the responses of patients to items rated as most often experienced and most important. The instrument has four scales:

- Parkinson symptoms, e.g. difficulties with writing; shuffling and difficulties getting up from a chair;
- Systemic symptoms, e.g. difficulties with walking; feeling generally unwell and feelings of extreme exhaustion;
- Emotional function, e.g. difficulties with concentration; difficulties accepting the disease; feeling depressed or discouraged;
- Social function, e.g. no longer able to do hobbies; illness inhibits sex life; difficulties with transport.

The instrument was tested for scaling by factor analysis, and tested for validity through correlations with patient-rated disease severity and other health status scores. The PDQL has been reported as predictive of patterns of use of health professionals by patients with PD.[23] In a community study of patients with PD in Wales significant associations were found between the Webster scale of disease severity and PDQL scores.[24]

The Parkinson's Disease Activities of Daily Living Scale

Hobson *et al.* developed an instrument, The Parkinson's Disease Activities of Daily Living Scale (PADLS) as a self-report scale of activities of daily living in PD.[25] The instrument was examined for reproducibility and then examined for validity through correlations with the PDQL, with depression scales and the Webster scale of disease severity.

The Parkinson's Disease Questionnaire

The Parkinson's Disease Questionnaire (PDQ-39) was developed through a series of exploratory open-ended interviews with patients with PD invited to describe the impact of the disease on their lives.[26] From analysis of these interviews a questionnaire with 65 items regarding different problems was drafted and sent to patients with PD in the community in England. Statistical analysis of results produced a shorter version (39 items), which was then sent to a further series of respondents along with other questionnaires to examine validity. A subsample completed two questionnaires over three to six days to test reproducibility. In addition, a further study of validity involved a clinic sample completing the 39-item version and SF-36 at two points over four months whilst also being assessed by neurologists with the Hoehn and Yahr and Columbia scales.[27] The resulting questionnaire comprises 39 items contributing to eight scales: mobility; activities of daily living; emotional well-being; stigma; social support; cognitions; communication; and bodily discomfort. Subsequent analyses have been used to produce a single summed index version of the instrument and also a shorter eight-item version, which can also be summed into a single index.[28,29] A subsequent community survey of individuals with PD showed that problems of access to services for PD was associated with poorer PDQ-39 scores.[30]

A number of studies have examined factors that might predict PDQ-39 scores. Lyons *et al.* examined components of the UPDRS and found that whilst postural and gait problems in the UPDRS were predictive of poorer PDQ-39 scores, other components such as rigidity and tremor were only weakly associated.[31] Other studies suggest that, as with the other health-related quality of life measures already discussed, depression is an important predictor of PDQ-39 scores; it often makes a greater contribution than either disease severity or disability.[32,33]

The evidence of the sensitivity to change and hence of appropriateness for evaluative studies of PDQ-39 is now very extensive. A number of observational longitudinal studies, both hospital-and community-based, with follow-up periods varying from four to

18 months, have shown significant changes over time in PDQ-39 reported by patients with PD.[27,34,35] In addition a number of intervention studies have observed significant changes over time in the instrument. Trials of cabergoline,[36] entacapone[37] and pergolide[38] have obtained significant changes over time in various dimensions of the PDQ-39. Renewed interest in neurosurgical interventions for PD has also resulted in studies showing marked improvements in PDQ-39 arising from pallidotomy[39,40] and deep-brain stimulation of the subthalamic nuclei.[41,42] Generally, there have been few evaluations of rehabilitation for PD using PDQ-39 as an outcome measure. An exception is a small study of an eight-week supervised exercise programme for PD which found significant improvements on PDQ-39 as well as the UPDRS.[43]

Utility or preference measures

A criticism of health-related quality of life measures has been that, whilst they may show the various gains and losses for different dimensions of health and healthcare, they do not provide an overall summary of the net or overall preference patients may have for given health states and health outcomes. Health economists have long maintained that patients' overall preferences need to be assessed by techniques that require that they judge 'preferences' for given health states against hypothetical risk or loss, for example financial loss or death. An early application of this approach to PD involved patients with PD rating their preferences for different stages of Hoehn and Yahr and different proportions of time spent in 'off' time.[44] The results were used to argue that although patients rated advanced stages of Hoehn and Yahr and high proportions of 'off' time quite negatively, they were overall risk averse, that is they would not undergo considerable risk of (hypothetical death) to stand a chance of avoiding such states.

This approach has not been extensively tested in PD. Formally it requires patients to make quite unusual and challenging judgements about the relative desirability of different health states; such judgements may be unfamiliar and difficult for older patients with PD. Instead studies have used health status instruments which other samples (non-PD) have rated for utilities and applied the numerical values to evaluate interventions for PD. Thus Gray *et al.* obtained significant improvements in this utility-based approach to health-related quality of life for patients undergoing pallidotomy.[40]

An instrument known as EQ-5D comprises a small number of simple questions about health status, to which utility values have been attached through respondents' ratings of the relative overall utility of different health states.[44]

> The EQ-5D has been shown to agree with PDQ-39, UPDRS and Hoehn and Yahr staging in a sample of patients with PD.[45]

Conclusions

There are now available well-established methods for evaluating outcomes of interventions for PD. In addition to validated clinical scales such as the UPDRS, there are a range of instruments providing evidence of outcomes from the patient's perspective. A number of analyses have demonstrated that the two sources provide important complementary evidence. The next step in this field is to gain a clearer understanding of the relative advantages of different measures. An example of the work now required is a study by Marinus *et al.* in which two independent reviewers examined available evidence for measurement properties of disease-specific health-related quality of life measures for PD.[46] They concluded that, whilst the selection of a measure will always depend on investigators' goals, nevertheless at present the PDQ-39 will probably be the most appropriate health-related quality of life measure. Other reviews have reached similar conclusions.[47,48]

Above all, given that neither drug- nor surgery-based interventions can be expected to completely solve the health problems of PD, it is essential that more evaluations of rehabilitation are conducted. In addition to the primary benefit of such studies in identifying effective interventions, it will be possible to perform more direct comparisons of outcome measures within studies to determine which measures are most appropriate for rehabilitation research. The patient's perspective regarding benefits of neurological rehabilitation is clearly distinctive from that obtained by conventional clinical assessment.[49] The vast majority of the evidence reviewed in this chapter has come from evaluations of drugs or neurosurgery, which may not necessarily generalize to the context of rehabilitation. There are also outstanding methodological issues regarding the capacity of the most frail and cognitively impaired to participate in self-assessing health status.

Note that it is beyond the scope of this chapter to consider measurement of outcomes on the carer of individuals with PD. However, it is clear that the carer's perspective is also distinctive and central. Overall there now exists a coherent framework within outcomes assessment to clearly guide the future evaluation of interventions for individuals with PD.

References

1 Hoehn M, Yahr M (1967) Parkinsonism: onset, progression and mortality. *Neurology* **17**: 427–42.

2. Martinez-Martin P (1993) Rating scales in Parkinson's disease. In: Jankovic J, Tolosa E, eds, *Parkinson's Disease and Movement Disorders*, 2nd ed. Williams and Wilkins, Baltimore: 281–92.

3. Fahn S, Elton R and members of the UPDRS Development Committee (1987) The Unified Parkinson's Disease Rating Scale. In: Fahn S, Marsden C, Calne D, Goldstein M, eds, *Recent Developments in Parkinson's Disease*. Macmillan Healthcare Information, Florham Park: 153–63.

4. van Hilten J, van der Zwan A, Zwinderman A, Roos R (1994) Rating impairment and disability in Parkinson's disease: evaluation of the Unified Parkinson's Disease Rating Scale. *Mov Disord* **9**: 84–8.

5. Mitchell S, Harper D, Lau A, Bhalla R (2000) Patterns of outcome measurement in Parkinson's disease clinical trials. *Neuroepidemiology* **19**: 100–8.

6. Welburn P, Walker S (1988) Assessment of quality of life in Parkinson's disease. In: Teeling-Smith G, *Measuring Health: A Practical Approach*. John Wiley & Son, London: 89–108.

7. Longstreth W, Nelson L, Linde M, Munoz D (1992) Utility of the Sickness Impact Profile in Parkinson's disease. *J Geriat Psychiatry Neurol* **5**: 142–8.

8. Martinez-Martin P, Frades Payo B and the Grupo Centro for the Study of Movement Disorders (1998) Quality of life in Parkinson's disease: validation study of the PDQ-39 Spanish version. *J Neurol* **245**(Suppl.): S34–S38.

9. Brown R, MacCarthy B, Jahanshahi M, Marsden D (1989) Accuracy of self-reported disability in patients with Parkinsonism. *Arch Neurol* **46**: 955–59.

10. Rothwell P, McDowell Z, Wong C, Dorman P (1997) Doctors and patients don't agree: cross-sectional study of patients' and doctors' perceptions and assessments of disability in multiple sclerosis. *BMJ* **314**: 1580–3.

11. Sprangers M, Aaronson N (1992) The role of health care providers and significant others in evaluating the quality of life of patients with chronic disease: a review. *J Clin Epidemiol* **45**: 743–60.

12. Hunt S McEwen J, McKenna S (1985) Measuring health status: a new tool for clinicians and epidemiologists. *J Roy Coll Gen Pract* **35**: 185–8.

13. Karlsen K, Larsen J, Tandberg E, Maeland J (1999) Influence of clinical and demographic variables on quality of life in patients with Parkinson's disease. *J Neurol Neurosurg Psychiatry* **66**: 431–5.

14. Karlsen K, Tandberg E, Arsland D, Larsen J (2000) Health-related quality of life in Parkinson's disease: a prospective longitudinal study. *J Neurol Neurosurg Psychiatry* **69**: 584–9.

15. Sitzia J, Haddrell V, Rice-Oxley M (1998) Evaluation of a nurse-led multidisciplinary neurological rehabilitation programme using the Nottingham Health Profile. *Clin Rehabil* **12**: 389–94.

16. Ware J, Sherbourne C (1992) The MOS 36-item short-form health survey (SF-36) I. Conceptual framework and item selection. *Med Care* **30**: 473–83.

17. Garratt A, Schmidt L, Mackintosh A, Fitzpatrick R (2002) Quality of life measurement: bibliographic study of patient assessed health outcome measures. *BMJ* **324**: 1417–19

18. Kuopio A, Marttila R, Helenius H *et al.* (2000) The quality of life in Parkinson's disease. *Mov Disord* **15**: 216–23.

19. Chrischilles E, Rubenstein L, Voelker M *et al.* (2002) Linking clinical variables to health-related quality of life in Parkinson's disease. *Parkinsonism Relat Disord* **8**: 199–209.

20. Gray A, McNamara I, Aziz T *et al.* (2002) Quality of life outcomes following surgical treatment of Parkinson's disease. *Mov Disord* **17**: 68–75.

21. Calne S, Schulzer M, Mak E *et al.* (1996) Validating a quality of life rating scale for idiopathic Parkinsonism: Parkinson's Impact Scale (PIMS). *Parkinsonism Relat Disord* **2**: 55–61.

22. De Boer A, Wijker W, Speelman J, de Haes J (1996) Quality of life in patients with Parkinson's disease: development of a questionnaire. *J Neurol Neurosurg Psychiatry* **61**: 70–4.

23. De Boer A, Sprangers M, Speelman H, de Haes H (1999) Predictors of health care use in patients with Parkinson's disease: a longitudinal study. *Mov Disord* **14**: 772–9.

24. Hobson P, Holden A, Meara J (1999) Measuring the impact of Parkinson's disease with the Parkinson's Disease Quality of Life questionnaire. *Age Ageing* **2**: 341–6.

25. Hobson J, Edwards N, Meara J (2001) The Parkinson's Disease Activities of Daily Living Scale: a new simple and brief measure of disability in Parkinson's disease. *Clin Rehabil* **15**: 241–6.

26. Peto V, Jenkinson C, Fitzpatrick R, Greenhall R (1995) The development and validation of a short measure of functioning and well-being for individuals with Parkinson's disease. *Qual Life Res* **4**: 241–8.

27. Fitzpatrick R, Peto V, Jenkinson C *et al.* Health-related quality of life in Parkinson's disease: a study of outpatient clinic attenders. *Mov Dis* **12**: 916–22.

28. Jenkinson C, Peto V, Fitzpatrick R *et al.* (1997) The Parkinson's Disease Questionnaire (PDQ-39): development and validation of a Parkinson's disease summary index score. *Age Ageing* **26**: 353–7.

29. Jenkinson C, Fitzpatrick R, Peto V, *et al.* (1997) The PDQ-8: development and validation of a short-form Parkinson's Disease Questionnaire. *Psychol Health* **12**: 805–14.

30. Peto V, Fitzpatrick R, Jenkinson C (1997) Self-reported health status and access to health services in a community sample with Parkinson's disease. *Disabil Rehabil* **19**: 97–103.

31. Lyons K, Pahwa R, Troster A, Koller W (1997) A comparison of Parkinson's disease symptoms and self reported functioning and well-being. *Parkinsonism Relat Disord* **3**: 207–9.

32. Schrag A, Jahanshahi M, Quinn N (2000) What contributes to quality of life in patients with Parkinson's disease? *J Neurol Neurosurg Psychiat* **69**: 308–12.

33. Global Parkinson's Disease Survey (GPDS) Steering Committee (2002) Factors impacting on quality of life in Parkinson's disease: results from an international survey. *Mov Disord* **17**: 6–67.

34. Harrison J, Preston S, Blunt S (2000) Measuring symptom change in patients with Parkinson's disease. *Age Ageing* **29**: 41–5.

35. Peto V, Jenkinson C, Fitzpatrick R (2001) Determining minimally important differences for the PDQ-39 Parkinson's Disease Questionnaire. *Age Ageing* **30**: 299–302.

36. Baas H, Shueler P (2001) Efficacy of cabergoline in long term use. *Eur Neurol* **46**: 18–23.

37. Durif F, Devaux I, Pere J *et al.* and the F-01 Study Group. (2001) Efficacy and tolerability of entacapone as adjunctive therapy to levodopa in patients with Parkinson's disease and end of dose deterioration in daily medical practice: an open multicenter study. *Eur Neurol* **45**: 111–28.

38. Koller W, Lees A, Doder M, Hely M and the Tolcapone/Pergolide Study Group (2001) Randomized trial of tolcapone versus pergolide as add-on to levodopa therapy in Parkinson's disease patients with motor-fluctuations. *Mov Disord* **16**: 858–66.

39. Martinez-Martin P, Valldeoriola F, Molinuevo J *et al.* (2000) Pallidotomy and quality of life in patients with Parkinson's disease: an early study. *Mov Disord* **15**: 65–70.

40. Gray A, McNamara I, Aziz T *et al.* (2002) Quality of life outcomes following surgical treatment of Parkinson's disease. *Mov Disord* **17**: 68–75.

41. Martinez-Martin P, Valldeoriola F, Tolosa E *et al.* (2002) Bilateral subthalamic nucleus stimulation and quality of life in advanced Parkinson's disease. *Mov Disord* **17**: 372–7.

42. Just H, Ostergaard K (2002) Health-related quality of life in patients with advanced Parkinson's disease treated with deep brain stimulation of the subthalamic nuclei. *Mov Disord* **17**: 539–45.

43. Baatile J, Langbein W, Weaver F *et al.* (2000) Effect of exercise on perceived quality of life of individuals with Parkinson's disease. *J Rehabil Res Dev* **37**: 529–34.

44. Brooks R (1996) EuroQol: the current state of play. *Health Policy* **37**: 53–72.

45. Schrag A, Selai C, Jahanshahi M, Quinn N (2000) The EQ-5D – a generic quality of life measure – is a useful instrument to measure quality of life in patients with Parkinson's disease. *J Neurol Neurosurg Psychiatry* **69**: 67–73.

46. Marinus J, Ramaker C, van Hilten J, Stiggelbout A (2002) Health-related quality of life in Parkinson's disease: a systematic review of disease-specific instruments. *J Neurol Neurosurg Psychiatry* **72**: 241–8.

47. Damiano A, Snyder C, Strausser B, Willian M (1999) A review of health-related quality of life concepts and measures for Parkinson's disease. *Qual Life Res* **8**: 235–43.

48. Gaudet P (2002) Measuring the impact of Parkinson's disease: an occupational therapy perspective. *Can J Occup Ther* **69**: 104–13.

49. Edwards S, Playford D, Hobart J, Thompson A (2002) Comparison of physician outcome measures and patients' perception of benefits of inpatient neurorehabilitation. *BMJ* **324**: 1493.

6

Future Directions: the Potential for Recovery and Repair

Simon JG Lewis and Roger A Barker

Introduction

Parkinson's disease (PD) is a common neurodegenerative disorder of the brain and typically presents with a disorder of movement. The core pathological event underlying the condition is the loss of the dopaminergic nigrostriatal pathway with the formation of α-synuclein-positive Lewy bodies. In the initial stages of the illness compensatory mechanisms exist that limit the extent of the dopaminergic loss but with time these fail and the disease becomes manifest. In this chapter we briefly outline the processes that underlie the innate plasticity of the adult CNS with respect to PD and how this may be exploited using neuroprotective and neurotrophic factors as well as curative cell therapies.

The core pathologically relevant degeneration of the nigrostriatal tract leads to the biochemical depletion of dopamine, most significantly in the posterolateral putamen,[1,2] which correlates with the degree of physical disability.[3] Therefore, given this, dopamine replacement has been the major treatment strategy. However, with time, L-dopa produces its own side-effects including 'on-off' phenomena – this has meant that the need for improved PD treatment continues to be of the utmost importance. Obviously, as with any disease, preventing patients from developing PD in the first instance would be the most desirable situation and in this respect understanding the processes underlying endogenous (innate) or exogenous (engineered) brain repair may be important. In this chapter we therefore explore this by discussing endogenous repair processes and the use of neuroprotective and cell replacement therapy.

Innate Plasticity in the Parkinsonian Brain

The adult CNS has long been thought of as being incapable of responding to damage or changes in sensory inputs. These concepts have had to be radically rethought over the last two decades following the pioneering work of Merzenich and colleagues in the adult mammalian somatosensory system. (This is reviewed in Buonomano and Merzenich.[4])

Cajal encapsulated the notion that the CNS is not capable of regeneration, 'Once development was ended, the founts of growth and regeneration of axons and dendrites dried up irrevocably. In adult centres, the nerve paths are something fixed and immutable; everything may die, nothing may be regenerated.'[5]

However, it is now recognized that the adult CNS shows a marked degree of plasticity and that this involves a number of processes including axonal sprouting, activation of silent synapses and the reorganization of pathways at the cortical and subcortical levels.[6]

The neurobiological basis of many of these changes are poorly understood, and the contribution of each process varies according to type and extent of the injury, especially given the diverse role of CNS glial cells as both mediators of CNS repair and inhibitors of regeneration.

However, with respect to the dopaminergic pathway, one important strategy is compensation. This describes the process that occurs over a period of time in which there is upregulation of the remaining dopaminergic system to take over the function of the lost neurones and thereby compensate for their loss. Clear experimental evidence for such a process has been identified after damage of forebrain dopamine systems in rats, provided that there is sparing of at least a few of the midbrain dopamine neurones that project to the striatum. The acute stage is followed by a period of recovery that can take place over a period of days, weeks and even months. These remaining neurones increase their synthesis and turnover of dopamine and by so doing promote the recovery of function.[7] In other words, the few remaining neurones undergo a dramatic upregulation that restores a similar level of dopaminergic tone in the striatum as was originally provided by the full normal population of neurones functioning at a lower level of neuronal activity and neurotransmitter turnover.

This compensation within a given biochemical pathway implies that there is considerable redundancy in the forebrain dopamine system, such that residual neurones are capable of compensating fully for up to 90–95% neuronal loss before permanent deficits are apparent. This is paralleled clinically in PD (Figure 6.1). In the human disease, symptoms are only apparent when the number of lost dopamine neurones exceeds 50%. At this stage of cell loss, dopamine replacement therapy is required and is effective. However, once the dopamine cell loss exceeds approximately 90%, then side-effects and other problems with the therapy arise, including the rapid switching of the patient from an 'on', often dyskinetic, state to an 'off' akinetic one. The similar ranges of depletions in the animal lesion and in the human disease suggest that in the early stages of PD plasticity of the spared neurones is fully able to compensate for the early cell loss. The symptoms then only

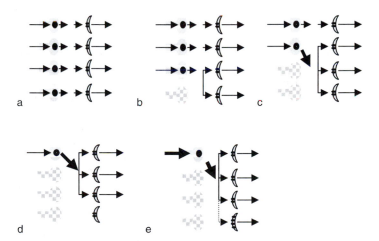

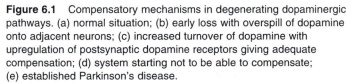

Figure 6.1 Compensatory mechanisms in degenerating dopaminergic pathways. (a) normal situation; (b) early loss with overspill of dopamine onto adjacent neurons; (c) increased turnover of dopamine with upregulation of postsynaptic dopamine receptors giving adequate compensation; (d) system starting not to be able to compensate; (e) established Parkinson's disease.

become apparent once the dopaminergic cell loss is already quite advanced. Thus, it is not that recovery cannot take place in chronic disease but rather that recovery is only able to keep pace with the slow progression of the disease up to a certain point. Once this critical point is reached the disease becomes manifest. Thereafter, the spontaneous compensation cannot keep up with the disease process, and the symptoms then become manifest.

In addition to these biochemical compensatory mechanisms at the level of the dopaminergic system, there is also evidence from rodent studies that the dopaminergic neuronal population may be constantly turning over in adult life. In other words, the loss of dopaminergic neurones, which occurs naturally with ageing, is matched by the local migration and differentiation of endogenous adult neural stem cells (NSCs). Until recently it was believed that the adult CNS was incapable of generating any new neurones, but it is now well known that adult NSCs are found at a number of CNS sites including the subventricular zone and dentate gyrus of the hippocampus.[8,9] Furthermore these cells have been identified in the adult human brain[10,11] and more recently in rodent studies these cells have been shown to become functionally integrated into host circuitry and mediate behavioural effects.[12–14] Furthermore these NSCs have been found to respond to a number of environmental and hormonal manipulations, although the significance of this is as yet unresolved.[15] Of interest in PD is the recent unpublished observations of Zhao *et al.* that the dopaminergic neurones of the rodent midbrain turnover in adult life.[16] This has led to the suggestion that such a mechanism may be defective in PD and contributing to disease progression and expression,[17] although it may also be viewed as being important in minimizing clinical expression early on in the course of the illness. Obviously further work is needed to address these issues but whatever the significance of this finding and hypothesis, it raises issues as to the role of endogenous NSCs in PD. This in turn has implications for developing repair strategies.

Strategies to Rescue the Dopaminergic System in Parkinson's Disease

Neuroprotection

Neuroprotection is a concept with broad applications across many neurodegenerative conditions. In relation to PD some claims of neuroprotection have already been made, most notably with the monoamine oxidase-B inhibitor selegiline. Interest in the neuroprotective capabilities of this drug stemmed from studies involving the 1-methyl-4-phenyl–1,2,3,6 tetrahydropyridine (MPTP) model of PD developed in the 1980s. In these early studies it was shown[18] both *in vitro* and *in vivo*, that the administration of selegiline protected dopaminergic neurones to MPTP toxicity, namely afforded a significant degree of neuroprotection. This was interpreted as a result of the monoamine oxidase enzyme being inhibited by selegiline and by so doing preventing the formation of the neurotoxic 1-methyl-4-phenylpyridinium ion (MPP+) from MPTP (but see also reference 19). These data were sufficiently robust to merit a prospective randomized, double-blind, placebo-controlled study evaluating the effect of selegiline on progression in early PD patients[20] on the basis that some environmental toxin similar to MPP+ may underlie the development of idiopathic PD. This study (the DATATOP study) demonstrated a significant delay in the deterioration of parkinsonian signs and symptoms in patients taking selegiline, as opposed to placebo or low-dose vitamin E. This suggested that the drug was having a neuroprotective action, although by virtue of its MAO inhibition it will have a symptomatic effect by inhibiting the breakdown of endogenously produced dopamine. Subsequent studies and analysis have confirmed that this is the mode of action, rather than a neuroprotective one. Nevertheless recent experiments have shown that, at least in laboratory models, selegiline may possess anti-apoptotic qualities, which may retard the cell loss in PD[21] and thus may still have some neuroprotective properties.

Other prospective neuroprotective agents that have been proposed in PD include the dopamine agonists[22] and anti-glutamatergic drugs.[23–25] No clinical studies have been reported to date that definitively confirm that dopamine agonists slow the disease process, although recent unpublished PET data are encouraging in this respect.[26] Certainly *in vitro*, dopamine agonists have been shown to protect embryonic dopaminergic neurones against a variety of toxins that may play a role in the development of the clinical condition.[27–29] This effect of dopamine agonists may be explained in terms of their known anti-oxidant effects.[30] A potential role for antiglutamatergic therapies in the neuroprotection of PD is also providing much interesting data. Increased glutamate release and subsequent excessive stimulation of the various glutamate receptors are thought to play critical roles in the pathophysiological mechanisms underlying many neurological diseases, including PD. It is well known that in PD the subthalamic nucleus, which provides widespread glutamate-mediated connections to various regions, is overactive. Agents that block glutamate release or act as glutamate receptor antagonists have been documented as protecting dopamine neurones from MPTP toxicity[31–33] and clinical trials are underway to explore their benefit further.

Neurotrophic factors

The use of neurotrophic factors to rescue populations of neurones has been widely explored for a number of years, although the translation from experimental studies to clinical trials has proven disappointing in a number of conditions including PD. The slow degeneration of dopaminergic neurones within the substantia nigra pars compacta (SNc) makes PD an attractive disorder for neurotrophic factor treatment. A large number of neurotrophic factors have been explored in PD[31] but most of the attention recently has concentrated on glial cell line-derived neurotrophic factor (GDNF). The discovery of the dopaminotrophic factor GDNF in 1993 led to a series of subsequent studies that have demonstrated that GDNF has both a neuroprotective and restorative capacity in animal models of PD.[32] However, intracerebroventricular GDNF administration in PD proved disappointing clinically and a single post-mortem case of a patient receiving such an infusion showed no evidence of dopaminergic cell rescue or fibre sprouting.[33] Alternative forms of GDNF delivery, such as through viral vectors or directly into the brain parenchyma,[34] may prove more effective, and clinical trials have recently commenced to investigate the intraparenchymal administration of GDNF in PD patients. Preliminary data from this trial suggest that GDNF delivered by such a route is effective both in terms of mediating a clinical response and in increasing dopaminergic innervation within the striatum as evidenced by fluorodopa PET scans.[35]

Strategies to Replace Dopamine Neurons in Parkinson's Disease

Human fetal allografts

An alternative experimental approach to treating PD is to try to actually repair the brain using neural tissue, most notably human embryonic dopaminergic nigral allografts. This approach has been developed clinically over the last 15 years, based on experimental work showing that embryonic dopaminergic cells harvested from the developing midbrain can be grafted and survive longterm in the adult CNS.[6,36] These grafts not only survive longterm but receive and make synapses with the host brain and restore a range of deficits in animal models of PD.[6,36–38]

Against this background, patients with advanced PD were first grafted with human embryonic tissue in the 1980s; over 300 such transplants have now been carried out. In many centres the results have been very encouraging with good clinical responses correlating well with longterm increased fluorodopa signal on PET scans (Figure 6.2) and restoration of normal activation of motor cortical areas.[6,36,39–42] Indeed, some patients with good clinical responses have come to post-mortem having unfortunately died, over a year after the procedure, from unrelated causes. In these cases there is clear evidence of surviving dopaminergic cells within the graft without evidence of any disease or rejection within the transplant.[43]

However, the procedure is not without controversy as was highlighted by the recent double-blind placebo-controlled study by Freed *et al*.[44] In this study 40 patients with advanced PD were randomized to receive either a graft of human embryonic nigral tissue or sham surgery, with the control arm being offered a graft at the end of one-year follow-up. Of the patients offered grafts in the control arm, only 14 were recruited because of concerns over the side-effects that had developed in some patients. These side-effects consisted of runaway dyskinesias and dystonia – defined as involuntary movements in the absence of any oral dopaminergic therapy. This occurred in five patients and was so severe in two that they required further neurosurgical intervention[45] and the conclusions drawn by some of the research team was that this approach cannot be recommended. However, nine of the patients did improve, especially those under the age of 60 years, and so the procedure was not without benefit in a significant number of patients as had been reported in other trials. Clearly it is important to know why the patients developed such disabling dyskinesias given that other groups have not seen such severe complications, although they have been reported to a lesser extent at least in the very well studied patients from Lund in Sweden.[46] Whilst it is not known why these patients developed these severe complications, it is important to note that the Freed *et al*. study was different from

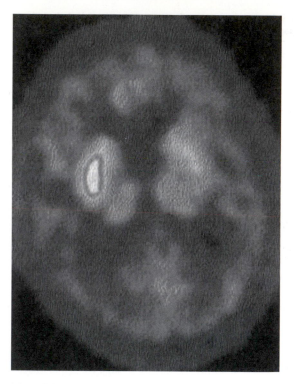

Figure 6.2   PET scan data showing PD patient with a unilateral graft of human embryonic tissue 10 years post implantation. The graft can clearly be seen whilst the patients own dopaminergic system has degenerated. Courtesy of Dr Paola Piccini, MRC Cyclotron Unit, Hammersmith Hospital, London.

others in a number of ways (Table 6.1) and some or none of these may have been important. One distinct possibility is that the patients chosen for grafting were more advanced and had a higher degree of drug-induced dyskinesia prior to transplantation or alternatively that the grafts were placed more ventrally within the striatal complex. Whatever the explanation, it is clear that this technique remains experimental and fraught with ethical and practical difficulties, especially given that this type of approach requires using aborted human fetal tissue. As a result other cells are being considered, including neural stem cells and xenografts.

Table 6.1 Fundamental differences in the Freed *et al.* study as compared to other published studies

TISSUE	Less tissue used per side of brain
	Tissue prepared and stored in a different way to other studies
	Tissue grafted using a novel transfrontal approach
PATIENT SELECTION	Possibly more advanced with greater dyskinesias pre-operatively
	No immunosuppression
TRIAL DESIGN	Sham surgery
	One-year follow-up with subjective primary end-point

Porcine neural xenografts

The difficulties with using human fetal tissue have led to the search for alternative sources of tissue, such as porcine neural cells. However, there are fundamental problems with using such tissue including risks of infection and issues of immune rejection.[47,48] Neither of these have been resolved experimentally and so it is not surprising that the clinical results to date have been largely disappointing with some clinical improvement but no significant dopaminergic cell survival at post-mortem or on fluorodopa PET scans.[49–51]

Neural stem cells

Neural stem cells (NSCs) can be found in the developing and adult brain and are capable of self-renewal for long periods of time, while retaining their ability to produce neurones, astrocytes and oligodendrocytes. (For reviews see references 9 and 52.) These features should render them suitable for replacement of neurones lost through injury or disease. Initial studies demonstrated that NSCs could be expanded from the rodent brain[53,54] and more recently from the developing human brain. This can be achieved using a novel passaging technique[55] or a combination of growth factors.[56–58] Recently it has been shown that significantly increased numbers of neurones can be generated from these cultures when maintaining cell-to-cell contact and neurotrophic factor treatment.[59]

However, despite the fact that large numbers of neurones can be obtained, there is yet no way of controlling their neurochemical phenotype as the major default pathway for neurones is GABA. This is a problem with regard to using these cells in PD where dopamine-producing neurones would be required. So is it possible to direct NSCs to become dopamine neurones?

Some studies have used epigenetic factors to induce tyrosine hydroxylase – a critical enzyme in normal dopamine synthesis – in rat- or mouse-derived neurospheres,[60–63] conditioned medium from a glial cell line,[64] or expanding cells under low oxygen conditions.[65] Two other studies have taken a more mechanistic approach using factors known to be important in dopaminergic neuronal development.[66,67]

Transplantation of NSCs into the brain has had varying results depending on the age of the host and the region into which the cells were grafted. Transplants into neurogenic regions of the adult brain resulted in differentiation of site-specific cells in the granular layer of the hippocampus and the olfactory bulb.[68,69] However, in non-neurogenic regions this is not the case. In addition, several studies demonstrate that many NPCs differentiate into astrocytes following transplantation.[70–73] These studies demonstrate that these cells can survive transplantation and hence may be a viable option for the treatment of PD. However, further techniques are required to produce dopamine neurones prior to transplantation and much work needs to be done to establish the functional effects of such transplants. Nevertheless anecdotal reports of successful stem cell transplants are beginning to be reported (MF Lévesque, presented at the American Association of Neurological Surgeons, 8 April 2002) although the basis for any benefit must remain conjectural at this stage given what is known experimentally with these cells.

Conclusions

Parkinson's disease is a common and complex disorder for which there is no obvious cause in the majority of cases. In the early stages, a number of compensatory mechanisms are recruited, which means that symptoms only appear after a number of years and a 50% loss of dopaminergic activity in the nigrostriatal pathway. The major compensatory pathway involves the dopaminergic neurones themselves but a possible role for NSCs has been suggested. As a result a number of strategies can be exploited including drugs to promote dopaminergic cell survival as well as cell replacement therapies. Most of these treatments remain unproven and/or experimental but may become more widely available in the future. We have discussed each of these strategies to highlight the range of approaches although other strategies are under active investigation, which we have not explored in this brief review, e.g. viral vectors and cell lines engineered to deliver trophic factors or dopamine. As to which approach will ultimately cure patients of PD is unknown but it is critical that we begin by better understanding the endogenous and exogenous reparative mechanisms of the parkinsonian brain.

Acknowledgements

The authors' own work is supported by the Parkinson's Disease Society and the MRC.

References

1. Kish SJ, Shannak K, Hornykiewicz O (1988) Uneven pattern of dopamine loss in the striatum of patients with idiopathic Parkinson's disease. Pathophysiologic and clinical implications. *N Engl J Med* **318**(14): 876–80.
2. Bernheimer H, Birkmayer W, Hornykiewicz O *et al.* (1973) Brain dopamine and the syndromes of Parkinson and Huntington. Clinical, morphological and neurochemical correlations. *J Neurol Sci* **20**(4): 415–55.
3. Morrish PK, Sawle GV, Brooks DJ (1996). Regional changes in [18F]dopa metabolism in the striatum in Parkinson's disease. *Brain* **119**: 2097–103.
4. Buonomano DV, Merzenich MM (1998) Cortical plasticity: from synapses to maps. *Annu Rev Neurosci* **21**: 149–86.
5. Cajal SR (1928) *Degeneration and Regeneration of the Nervous System*. Oxford University Press, Oxford.
6. Barker RA; Dunnett SB (1999) *Neural Repair, Transplantation and Rehabilitation*. Psychology Press, Hove.
7. Zigmond MJ, Abercrombie ED, Berger TW, *et al.* (1990) Compensations after lesions of central dopaminergic neurons: some clinical and basic implications. *Trends Neurosci* **13**(7): 290–6.
8. Armstrong RJ, Svendsen CN (2000) Neural stem cells: from cell biology to cell replacement. *Cell Transplant* **9**(2): 139–52.
9. Gage FH (2001) Mammalian neural stem cells. *Science* **287**: 1433–8.

10. Eriksson PS, Perfilieva E, Bjork-Eriksson T, *et al.* (1998) Neurogenesis in the adult human hippocampus. *Nat Med* **4**(11): 1313–17.

11. Johansson CB, Svensson M, Wallstedt L *et al.* (1999) Neural stem cells in the adult human brain. *Exp Cell Res* **253**(2): 733–6.

12. Shors TJ, Miesegaes G, Beylin A *et al.* (2001) Neurogenesis in the adult is involved in the formation of trace memories. *Nature* **410**(6826): 372–6.

13. Song HJ, Stevens CF, Gage FH (2002). Neural stem cells from adult hippocampus develop essential properties of functional CNS neurons. *Nat Neurosci* **5**(5): 438–45.

14. Carlen M, Cassidy RM, Brismar H *et al.* (2002) Functional integration of adult-born neurons. *Curr Biol* **12**(7): 606–8.

15. Van Praag H, Kempermann G, Gage FH (2000) Neural consequences of environmental enrichment. *Nat Rev Neurosci* **1**(3): 191–8.

16. Zhao M, Momma S, Delfabi K *et al.* (2000) Demonstration of tyrosine-hydroxylase positive apoptotic neurons in adult substantia nigra although total nigral neuronal numbers remain constant during the life span of male C57BL/6 mice. *Soc Neurosci* Abstract A114.1.

17. Armstrong RJ, Barker RA (2001) Neurodegeneration: a failure of neuroregeneration? *Lancet* **358**(9288): 1174–6.

18. Mytilineou C, Cohen G (1985) Deprenyl protects dopamine neurons from the neurotoxic effect of 1-methyl–4-phenylpyridinium ion. *J Neurochem* **45**(6): 1951–3.

19. Ebadi M, Sharma S, Shavali S, El Refaey H (2002) Neuroprotective actions of selegiline. *J Neurosci Res* **67**(3): 285–9.

20. Olanow CW, Hauser RA, Gauger L *et al.* (1995) The effect of deprenyl and levodopa on the progression of Parkinson's disease. *Ann Neurol* **38**(5): 771–7.

21. Tatton NA, Maclean-Fraser A, Tatton WG *et al.* (1998) A fluorescent double-labeling method to detect and confirm apoptotic nuclei in Parkinson's disease. *Ann Neurol* **44**(3 Suppl. 1): S142–S148.

22. Olanow CW, Jenner P, Brooks D (1988) Dopamine agonists and neuroprotection in Parkinson's disease. *Ann Neurol* **44**(3 Suppl. 1): S167–S174.

23. Turski L, Bressler K, Rettig KJ *et al.* (1991) Protection of substantia nigra from MPP+ neurotoxicity by N-methyl-D-aspartate antagonists. *Nature* **349**(6308): 414–18.

24. Barneoud P, Mazadier M, Miquet JM *et al.* (1996) Neuroprotective effects of riluzole on a model of Parkinson's disease in the rat. *Neuroscience* **74**(4): 971–83.

25. Boireau A, Dubedat P, Bordier F *et al.* (1994) Riluzole and experimental parkinsonism: antagonism of MPTP-induced decrease in central dopamine levels in mice. *Neuroreport* **5**(18): 2657–60.

26. Whone AL, Remy P, Davis MR *et al.* (2002) The REAL-PET study: slower progression in early Parkinson's disease treated with ropinirole compared with L-dopa. American Academy of Neurology Annual Meeting Abstract S11.006.

27. Carvey PM, Pieri S, Ling ZD (1997) Attenuation of levodopa-induced toxicity in mesencephalic cultures by pramipexole. *J Neural Transm* **104**(2–3): 209–28.

28. Sawada H, Ibi M, Kihara T *et al.* (1998) Dopamine D2-type agonists protect mesencephalic neurons from glutamate neurotoxicity: mechanisms of neuroprotective treatment against oxidative stress. *Ann Neurol* **44**(1): 110–119.

29. Gassen M, Gross A, Youdim MB (1998) Apomorphine enantiomers protect cultured pheochromocytoma (PC12) cells from oxidative stress induced by H_2O_2 and 6-hydroxydopamine. *Mov Disord* **13**(4): 661–7.

30. Nishibayashi S, Asanuma M, Kohno M *et al.* (1996) Scavenging effects of dopamine agonists on nitric oxide radicals. *J Neurochem* **67**(5): 2208–11.

31. Bradford HF, Zhou J, Pliego-Rivero B *et al.* (1999) Neurotrophins in the pathogenesis and potential treatment of Parkinson's disease. *Adv Neurol* **80**: 19–25.

32. Barker RA, Hurelbrink CB (2001) Prospects for the treatment of Parkinson's disease using neurotrophic factors. *Expert Opin Pharmacother* **2**(10): 1531–43.

33. Kordower JH, Palfi S, Chen EY *et al.* (1999) Clinicopathological findings following intraventricular glial-derived neurotrophic factor treatment in a patient with Parkinson's disease. *Ann Neurol* **46**(3): 419–24.

34. Kordower JH, Emborg ME, Bloch J *et al.* (2000) Neurodegeneration prevented by lentiviral vector delivery of GDNF in primate models of Parkinson's disease. *Science* **290**(5492): 767–73.

35. Gill S, Patel NK, O'Sullivan K *et al.* (2002) Intraparenchymal Putaminal Administration of Glial Derived Neurotrophic Factor in the Treatment of Advanced Parkinson's Disease. American Academy of Neurology Annual Meeting Abstract S31.003.

36. Freeman TB, Widner H, eds (1998) *Cell Transplantation for Neurological Disorders: Toward reconstruction of the human central nervous system.* Humana Press, New Jersey.

37. Dunnett SB, Everitt BJ (1998) Topographic factors affecting the functional viability of dopamine-rich grafts in the neostriatum. In: Freeman TB, Widner H, eds. *Cell Transplantation for Neurological Disorders: Toward reconstruction of the human central nervous system.* Humana Press, New Jersey: 135–169.

38. Björklund A, Dunnett SB, Stenevi U *et al.* (1980) Reinnervation of the denervated striatum by substantia nigra transplants: functional consequences as revealed by pharmacological and senorimotor testing. *Brain Res* **199**: 307–33.

39. Olanow CW, Kordower JH, Freeman TB (1996) Fetal nigral transplantation as a therapy for Parkinson's disease. *Trends Neurosci* **19**(3): 102–9.

40. Lindvall O (1997) Neural transplantation: a hope for patients with Parkinson's disease. *Neuroreport* **8**(14): 3–12.

41. Piccini P, Lindvall O, Björklund A *et al.* (2000) Delayed recovery of movement-related cortical function in Parkinson's disease after striatal dopaminergic grafts. *Ann Neurol* **48**(5): 689–95.

42. Piccini P, Brooks DJ, Bjorklund A *et al.* (1999) Dopamine release from nigral transplants visualized in vivo in a Parkinson's patient. *Nat Neurosci* **2**(12): 1137–40.

43. Kordower JH, Freeman TB, Olanow CW (1998) Neuropathology of fetal nigral grafts in patients with Parkinson's disease. *Mov Disord* **13**(Suppl. 1): 88–95.

44. Freed CR, Greene PE, Breeze RE *et al.* (2001) Transplantation of embryonic dopamine neurons for severe Parkinson's disease. *N Engl J Med* **344**(10): 710–9.

45. Olanow CW, Freeman T, Kordower J (2001) Transplantation of embryonic dopamine neurons for severe Parkinson's disease. *N Engl J Med* **345**(2): 146.

46. Widner H. The Lund Transplant Program for Parkinson's Disease and Patients with MPTP-Induced Parkinsonism. In: Freeman TB, Widner H, eds. *Cell Transplantation for Neurological Disorders: Toward reconstruction of the human nervous system.* Humana Press, New Jersey: 1–17.

47. Barker RA (2000) Porcine neural xenografts: what are the issues? *Novartis Found Symp* **231**: 184–96.

48. Barker RA, Kendall AL, Widner H (2000) Neural tissue xenotransplantation: what is needed prior to clinical trials in Parkinson's disease? Neural Tissue Xenografting Project. *Cell Transplant* **9**(2): 235–46.

49. Schumacher JM, Ellias SA, Palmer EP *et al.* (2000) Transplantation of embryonic porcine mesencephalic tissue in patients with PD. *Neurology* **54**(5): 1042–50.

50. Deacon T, Schumacher J, Dinsmore J *et al.* (1997) Histological evidence of fetal pig neural cell survival after transplantation into a patient with Parkinson's disease. *Nat Med* **3**(3): 350–3.

51. Hauser RA, Watts R, Freeman TB (2001) A double-blind, randomised, controlled, multicenter clinical trial of the safety and efficacy of transplanted fetal porcine ventral mesencephalic cells versus imitation surgery in patients with Parkinson's disease. *Mov Disord* **16**: 3–4.

52. McKay R (2000) Stem cells and the cellular organization of the brain. *J Neurosci Res* **59**(3): 298–300.

53. Gensburger C, Labourdette G, Sensenbrenner M (1987) Brain basic fibroblast growth factor stimulates the proliferation of rat neuronal precursor cells in vitro. *FEBS Letters* **217**(1): 1–5.

54. Reynolds BA, Tetzlaff W, Weiss S (1992) A multipotent EGF-responsive striatal embryonic progenitor cell produces neurons and astrocytes. *Journal of Neurosci* **12**(11): 4565–74.

55. Svendsen CN, ter Borg MG, Armstrong RJ *et al.* A new method for the rapid and long term growth of human neural precursor cells. *J Neurosci Methods* **85**: 141–52.

56. Vescovi AL, Parati EA, Gritti A *et al.* (1999) Isolation and cloning of multipotential stem cells from the embryonic human CNS and establishment of transplantable human neural stem cell lines by epigenetic stimulation. *Exp Neurol* **156**: 71–83.

57. Carpenter MK, Cui X, Hu Z-Y *et al.* In vitro expansion of a multipotent population of human neural progenitor cells. *Exp Neurol* **158**: 265–78.

58. Quinn SM, Walters WM, Vescovi AL, Whittemore SR (1999) Lineage restriction of neuroepithelial precursor cells from fetal human spinal cord. *J Neurosci Res* **57**: 590–602.

59. Caldwell MA, He X, Wilkie N, *et al.* (2001) Growth factors regulate the survival and fate of cells derived from human neurospheres. *Nat Biotechnol* **19**(5): 475–9.

60. Ling Z-D, Potter ED, Lipton JW, Carvey PM (1997). Differentiation of mesencephalic progenitor cells into dopaminergic neurons by cytokines. *Exp Neurol* **149**: 411–23.

61. Takahashi J, Palmer TD, Gage FH (1999) Retinoic acid and neurotrophins collaborate to regulate neurogenesis in adult-derived neural stem cell cultures. *J Neurobiol* **38**(1): 65–81.

62. Sanchez-Pernaute R, Studer L, Bankiewicz KS *et al.* (2001) In vitro generation and transplantation of precursor-derived human dopamine neurons. *J Neurosci Res* **65**(4): 284–8.

63. Stull ND, Jung JW, Iacovitti L (2001) Induction of a dopaminergic phenotype in cultured striatal neurons by bone morphogenetic proteins. *Brain Res Dev Brain Res* **130**(1): 91–8.

64. Daadi M, Weiss S (1999) Generation of tyrosine hydroxylase-producing neurons from precursors of the embryonic and adult brain. *J Neurosci* **19**(11): 4484–97.

65. Studer L, Csete M, Lee SH *et al.* (2000) Enhanced proliferation, survival, and dopaminergic differentiation of CNS precursors in lowered oxygen. *J Neurosci* **20**(19): 7377–83.

66. Sakurada K, Ohshima-Sakurada M, Palmer TD, Gage FH (1999) Nurr 1, an orphan nuclear receptor, is a transcriptional activator of endogenous tyrosine hydroxylase in neural progenitor cells derived from the adult brain. *Development* **126**(18): 4017–26.

67. Wagner J, Akerud P, Castro DS *et al.* (1999) Induction of midbrain dopaminergic phenotype in Nurr1 – overexpressing neural stem cells by type1 astrocytes. *Nature Biotechnol* **17**: 653–9.

68. Suhonen JO, Peterson DA, Ray J, Gage FH (1996). Differentiation of adult hippocampus-derived progenitors into olfactory neurons in vitro. *Nature* **383**: 624–7.

69. Fricker RA, Carpenter MK, Winkler C, *et al.* (1999) Site-specific migration and neuronal differentiation of human neural progenitor cells after transplantation in the adult rat brain. *J Neurosci* **19**(14): 5990–6005.

70. Svendsen CN, Clarke DJ, Rosser AE, Dunnett SB (1996) Survival and differentiation of rat and human epidermal growth factor-responsive precursor cells following grafting into the lesioned adult central nervous system. *Exp Neurol* **137**: 376–88.
71. Svendsen CN, Caldwell MA, Shen J *et al.* Long term survival of human central nervous system progenitor cells transplanted into a rat model of Parkinson's disease. *Exp Neurol* **148**(1): 135–46.
72. Winkler C, Fricker RA, Gates MA *et al.* (1998) Incorporation and glial differentiation of mouse EGF-responsive neural progenitor cells after transplantation into the embryonic rat brain. *Mol Cell Neurosci* **11**(3): 99–116.
73. Shihabuddin LS, Horner PJ, Ray J, Gage FH (2000) Adult spinal cord stem cells generate neurons after transplantation in the adult dentate gyrus. *J Neurosci* **20**(23): 8727–35.

Index

Page numbers in *italics* indicate figures or tables.